Far Away Cows

A Book About Cows, Engineers and Research Into Parkinson's Disease

Dr. Dario Toncich

First Edition Published 2004 by Chrystobel Engineering Publishers, Brighton
Australia

ISBN:1492896101
ISBN-13:9781492896104

"I shall be telling this with a sigh
Somewhere ages and ages hence:
Two roads diverged in a wood, and I –
I took the one less traveled by,
And that has made all the difference…"

-Robert Frost (1920)

CONTENTS

ACKNOWLEDGMENTS

This book is not a research book but, rather, a personal account of the unusual sorts of things that happen during the course of research and life. For this reason, the authorship of this book doesn't reflect the actual research contributions that are described herein, and this needs to be clarified from the outset.

My contribution to this research was to act as one of two supervisors for a doctoral research project in the area of Parkinson's Disease (PD). The doctoral research program that is described in this book was undertaken by our research candidate, Shahriar Yousefi, who deserves the credit for any specific contributions to the field that were made as a result. Credit is also due to Dr. Mark Schier, who co-supervised the project and provided the intellectual input in the areas of sensory neurosciences and psychophysiology. In so far as the general information pertaining to PD research is concerned, what is presented herein is only my interpretation of the thousands of person-years of work in the field, as carried out by other scientists and published in numerous journals and Internet sites.

For ethical reasons, it is not possible to thank (by directly naming) those people who were afflicted with PD and somehow managed to put that to one side in order to contribute their time to the research project described herein. Thanks are also due to our state-based Parkinson's support organization, who assisted us in our research and in the recruitment of participants who were afflicted with PD.

Dr. Dario Toncich

FOREWORD

If you have gotten to this page, you are probably wondering what cows, engineers and research into Parkinson's Disease all have in common. Superficially, one would think nothing at all.

However, if you choose to read on then you may discover, as I did, that in life strange bedfellows can often conspire to create interesting but true stories. This is one such story, and it took place over several years. Not – as C.S. Lewis once wrote – "*when your grandfather was a boy*" but, rather, quite recently. In this book, you have a chance to read a story that was written largely as it was happening.

In essence, this is a book about what happens along the much clichéd "*road less travelled*", and when engineers travel upon that road and become involved in things about which they know very little – that is, Parkinson's Disease and research into that disease. If you don't have Parkinson's Disease or have never come across it, then when you finish reading this, I hope that you may know something more about it, and how much it impacts upon the many people who do have it. If you are one of the many people in the world who do have Parkinson's Disease, then I hope you will one day forgive all engineers for my intrusion, and come to learn why we probably aren't the best people to choose to do research in the field. In either event, I hope that by reading this book you will ultimately come to understand what cows, engineers and research into Parkinson's Disease all have in common.

Dr. Dario Toncich

1 FROM COWS TO PARKINSON'S RESEARCH

When I was but 11 years of age, I was in the fifth grade of a Catholic school. It was there that my teacher, Sister Kevin, a dedicated and hard-nosed Irish nun, one day told me that I should never forget that *"far away cows have long horns"*. And, I never did.

Of course, at the time, I had no idea what Sister Kevin was talking about but I figured that, being saintly and sage-like, her cow philosophy would have important ramifications for the rest of my life – a compass if you will. Having been brought up in the city, and never having had much to do with cows, I elevated her cow reasoning to a higher plane, and assumed that this was sound advice for life, but not as I then knew it.

Sister Kevin, however, appeared to be relatively old – from the perspective of an 11-year-old, she looked to be over 150 but, in retrospect, she was probably only in her 50s. Nevertheless, given her perceived age, I had, on earlier occasions, dared to question some of her other philosophies, much to my chagrin. One of her other great pieces of reasoning related not to cows but, rather, to grades. She had told the class that she never gave out "A" grades because an "A" meant that we were perfect, and only God was perfect. The highest grade she could ever give, she said, was a "B".

Now, even at the age of 11, I could reason that if the highest grade that could be given was a "B", this would mean that anyone who got a "B" was perfect, and only God was perfect – how could this be? When I tried to explain this to her, I was met with the cantankerous Irish nun glare that was traditionally reserved to ward off blasphemers from further punitive action. I also quickly realized that if we pursued this argument through to its logical conclusion then, by the time we got to the grade of "Z", we would have consumed an entire alphabet – and, since only God was perfect, even a grade of "Z" would still be far too good.

I tell you all these things only because we may need to revisit them during the course of this book and because, if you choose to fault my reasoning, then you will ultimately come to understand, as Sister Kevin did, that I should only get a grade of "B", or less, for what is written herein.

I also need to explain to you how I got from the fifth grade, and spring-boarded from Sister Kevin's cow philosophy, to the dizzying heights of research mediocrity in engineering – and, even more strangely, from this, to become involved in research in the area of Parkinson's Disease (abbreviated as "PD"). If you have the patience to read these few pages, which will give you this background, you may come to a better understanding of the central theme of this book and its relevance. You may also come to understand my writing style, and learn to take what follows in the spirit in which it was intended.

In assembling this book, I had contemplated filling in my intermediate years in the tradition of *The Diary of Anne Frank*. So, I scoured my previous diaries for inspiration. Alas, an engineer's diary life does tend to lack some of the drama and passion required to sustain an audience. Two milestone entries in my former diaries included:

"Change cat's flea collar"

and

"Garbage day has moved to Tuesday."

Another annual milestone entry, which occurred each November, was:

"Buy new diary today".

I won't regale you with the less interesting entries but you can see that, with a life that had been as full and rich as this, it was self-evident that any treatise, based upon the intimate journal entries of an engineer, was unlikely to provide significant competition for Anne Frank's diary. For this reason, you will have to make do with an abridged version, as per my recollections.

Perhaps, I should start by explaining the force that drove me from the cow philosophy of the fifth grade to scientific and engineering disciplines. As you may be aware, engineering is predominantly a mathematics and physics-based discipline, so you could be forgiven for thinking that I was inspired by the likes of Einstein, Gödel and Fermi – but you would be very wrong.

In fact, my decision to pursue science and engineering was more to do with being an early-onset television addict, and my enduring admiration for the *Professor* on *Gilligan's Island*, which was highly popular on television during the 1960s. One had to have great respect for any individual who could make radio batteries out of coconut shells, and who took an entire chemistry laboratory set (and library of text books) with him on a *three hour tour*....

My other early scientific role model was *Dr. Zachary Smith* from the television series *Lost in Space*. Here was a Doctor of Inter-galactic Space Science with whom any aspiring 11 year old scientist could readily relate. He was one of very few male television characters in the 1960s who had enough intelligence to scream hysterically and run whenever confronted by an enormous, latex-covered, alien life-form that had been actuated by visible strings, dangling from the orange-painted sky on the set. Finally, a career scientist who reacted the way that I would have reacted in the same situation.

Of course, I did also have a more realistic role model – Professor Julius Sumner Miller, the American physicist, come television icon of the 1950s, 1960s and 1970s. Sumner Miller was the quintessential *mad scientist* that mesmerized children in the United States, Britain, Canada and Australia with his crazy physics experiments and with his incessant questioning of *"Why is it so?"* A cross between Albert Einstein and Jimmy Cagney, he managed to terrorize, amuse and, above all, fascinate anyone who was game to watch or participate in his television shows. My most enduring recollection of Sumner Miller was from one of his 1970s television shows (*The Professor and the Enquiring Minds*) where he performed an experiment and then bombastically yelled out to his high school participants,

"I'm gonna do it again! I'm gonna do it again! – Why?"

"To see if the results are repeatable?" asked one student.

"No! No! No!"

"To see if the results are accurate?" asked another.

"No! No! No! Why am I doing it again? Because I LIKE IT! Because I L I K E I T!" he roared, with an enthusiasm bordering on mania.

And that summed him up – a person who sought to inspire by telling the young that physics and science, like life, were meant to be full of fun and adventure and passion. As an individual with professorial chairs at universities in both California and New South Wales, Sumner Miller was prepared to do whatever it took to inspire young people to look at science, whether it was by playing the role of the crazy scientist in the *Frightenstein* television series in Canada, or appearing as the scientific clown on the Johnny Carson show in the United States, or as the *Kitchen Professor* in Australia. Sumner Miller drew millions of children around the world into the realms of science, and I was one of them.

With role models such as these, my high school and university paths had mapped themselves out and, some years later, I found myself holding on to a university degree in electrical engineering. Now, you may still be wondering, how did someone with an engineering degree get involved in an area of research such as PD, which is surely in the province of medical research? I will eventually get to this, albeit through a convoluted and torturous path, which will expose you to the cruel realities of a life encapsulated in an engineering persona.

By way of background, I suppose that you need to understand that engineers had already made significant contributions to various medical areas. For one thing, you may be aware that engineers had developed the world's first, truly effective contraceptive – their personality. Yes, I know it's an old line but, believe it or not, we engineers are perceived, by some, to be extremely dull people – you may refer back to my earlier diary highlights if you require further evidence.

I only discovered what people really thought of engineers after graduating, when I learnt that any party conversation could be immediately killed with a few choice words,

"...actually, I'm an engineer."

Generally, this declaration was sufficient to stun the recipient more effectively than a native's curare-filled blow-dart, and leave them desperately searching for a response. To the untrained eye, the glazed look on a recipient's face would appear to be a drug-induced coma but, to an engineer, it was the unmistakable symptom of a non-engineer trying to escape what they perceived to be an impending and excruciatingly boring dialogue.

I soon learnt to refer to this comatose state as *Easter Island Syndrome* because the recipients of *"...actually, I'm an engineer"* took on the stone-faced, taciturn expressions of the statues on the island of the same name. I also learnt that one was more likely to get a dialogue going with one of the Easter Island statues than with the recipient of *"actually, I'm an engineer"*.

Most people have no idea what engineers do, so tact generally forces them into a follow up question of:

"Can you fix a TV set?" and/or "Can you fix a car?"

which is the sum total of what they perceive engineering to be about. The millisecond or two that it takes an engineer to respond with a "No" leaves sufficient pause in the conversation to enable the stunned victim to shift their Easter Island gaze to another portion of the party room and then excuse themselves because they suddenly recognize someone else that they know and urgently have to talk to – they'll be right back a little later (and, of course, later never comes).

The most disturbing part of all of this is that we engineers can look around the same party room and hear people saying *"...actually, I'm a doctor"*, and can watch the recipient's eyes light up before they respond with *"how fascinating..."* as an opening to an ongoing dialogue.

I can also tell you that, not long after getting my first degree in engineering, I was working at the University of Melbourne, and coming home one evening, only to find that all the roads in the central business district had been cordoned off. This was part of a major security net for what was a Commonwealth Heads of Government (CHOGM) meeting at the Melbourne Town Hall. As there was no alternative but to walk, I wandered past the Town Hall, only to find that a meeting had just ended and some of the delegates had come out to do a *meet and greet*. As it turned out, I was coincidentally standing in front of one of the barricades when Indira Gandhi came out and decided to shake hands with me. Now, in the three seconds that we meaningfully interacted, I cannot honestly remember saying to her, *"...actually, I'm an engineer"* but I can report that, only a few months later, Indira Gandhi was gunned down and assassinated. As an engineer and a guilt-ridden Catholic, one can't help but feeling some sense of responsibility, thinking that she might have gone willingly to her death, just to avoid having to have any further dialogues with engineers that awaited her in *meet and greet* sessions.

In order to understand why we engineers are what we are, you also need to know a few other things about us, apart from our unmistakable charm. There are a few rules with which all engineers have been genetically programmed:

1.   *Never read instruction manuals – these are only for non-engineers*

2.   *Never read roadmaps – these are only for non-engineers*

3.   *Pay no attention to any object or living thing that can't be wound, cranked, started with a battery, or controlled with a keyboard, cell-phone or infra-red remote control*

4.   *If it has buttons, always push them, even if you don't know what they do*

5.   *If it doesn't work, hit it. If it still doesn't work, hit it harder. If it still doesn't work, it probably wasn't designed by an engineer and isn't worthy of our attention*

6.   *Art is really only framed wallpaper (refer back to Rule 3) – if God had really meant for people to paint, he wouldn't have created digital cameras and image processing software*

7.   *Literature is really only a textual form of art which is only framed wallpaper (refer back to Rule 3).*

As scientists unravel the human genetic code, there is no doubt in my mind that they will discover that we engineers fundamentally differ from other humans in the "*Gee, I wonder what happens when you push this button*" gene department.

I also need to warn you that we engineers don't communicate with one another (or with humans) in a manner to which people may be accustomed. Firstly, we can split an infinitive faster than a scientist can split an atom. More importantly, however, we engineers have evolved in such a way that we communicate and express emotion through a complicated language, which is composed of sarcastic comments; poisonous barbs; insults, and generally abusive or tasteless/insensitive derogatory remarks. This form of communication serves us well when dealing with emotionless electronic or mechanical devices – or, indeed, other engineers. However, as you will discover when you read through this book, it does tend to create problems on those rare occasions that we engineers have to interact with humans. This book is about many such occasions.

And, now that you understand the basic ground rules and genetics, you probably require a good *for-instance* to fully put you in touch with the engineering persona. To this end, I can tell you that my very first encounter with real engineers actually occurred before I got my engineering degree. And, yes, like many of you non-engineers, I too developed acute *Easter Island Syndrome* on my early encounters. My first experience with engineers occurred when I was employed, during my undergraduate years, by one of the local television networks, to develop a computer controlled tracking system for their electronic news gathering. One would imagine that, for an early-onset television addict, such an appointment would be akin to letting a child loose in a toy store, but I soon discovered that such organizations weren't as glamorous as one would expect.

The first thing that shocked me upon arrival was that the television world was divided into two distinct species – *on-air talent* and *off-air talent*. I observed that the way to tell them apart was the fact that the *on-air talent* was of average, or above average, appearance, whereas the *off-air talent* had appearances that would drive an *ugly-meter* deep into the red zone whenever it was pointed at them. There were clearly very, very good reasons why the *off-air talent* was kept *off-air* in commercial television networks. Did these *off-air* people take ugly-pills and put on fright wigs when they got out of bed in the morning, I wondered? Or was this some sort of subconscious rebellion against the superficiality of the appearance of the *on-air* talent? Maybe just looking at the *off-air* people gave the *on-air* people a greater sense of self-esteem about their own appearance, and allowed them to go about their business with more confidence than they otherwise might have had.

In any case, once I got over the shock of seeing what the *off-air talent* looked like, I also learnt that the *off-air talent* was divided into three groups (business, artistic and engineering) and that these were the basis of warring tribes that fired poisoned arrows at each other at every available opportunity.

On the whole, it appeared to me that the television world had made a very wise decision in putting business people in charge of a television network, despite the fact that these business people seemed to have no understanding or appreciation of either artistic or engineering matters, in an industry whose core business was founded on the selling of a combination of artistic and engineering matters.

Even at my tender age of 20, I could see that putting the artists in control would have led to certain bankruptcy because there would have been uncontrolled expenditure with no focus on income. Putting the engineers in charge would have led to controlled expenditure and certain bankruptcy because the program material would be so dull that nobody would watch. The only solution was to be management driven, thereby creating a triangle of suspicion, tension and brinkmanship between the tribes – which, in all fairness, appeared to working reasonably well when I arrived on the scene.

This management triangle quickly taught me that we engineers were not only dull but that we didn't even know how to fight very well. It's one thing to be dull, but quite another not to be able to fight off those artistic types who accuse you of being dull. In the brutal combat of the television environment, tribal clashes between engineers and artists would invariably lead to artists demanding that engineers deliver some silly device or technology that the engineers thought was either frivolous, costly or technically infeasible. Both tribes would prepare their weapons to fire into the management camp. The engineers would present a thick document, filled with technical details and costings. The artists would simply march into management; burst into tears; hold their breath; stamp their feet on the floor, and emerge minutes later having gained everything that they had wanted – hang the expense. One soon learnt that facts and technical details were simply no defense against the brutal assault of tears and foot stamping tantrums.

The real problem was self-evident – we engineers simply weren't genetically programmed for this kind of warfare – many of us were prepared to accept utter defeat and humiliation over the prospect of a display of tears, breath-holding and foot-stamping.

The commercial television network was my first ever job and, I have to say, it was quite a learning experience in more than just an engineering sense. For the first week of work, I had to report to the head of the engineering tribe. This gave me great insight into the engineering personality. For one thing, every morning when the head walked into the office, he asked me how I was, and then proceeded to slam the door right in my face before I had a chance to respond. Behind the door, I could hear the muffled sound of him saying,

"Good. Fine. Glad to hear it. Keep up the good work."

Noel Coward once said that his definition of a boor was any person who, when asked how they were, proceeded to tell you. Obviously the head of engineering was a fan of Coward – I figured, being in the television business, why shouldn't he be.

The more traumatic part of my brief time in the industry, however, came when I was told that I would be working with *Bill*, and that I would be sharing *Bill's Office*, and that I could move into *Bill's Office* immediately because he was on vacation. This sounded harmless enough until I introduced myself to people around the station and proudly informed them that I would be sharing *Bill's Office*. Every time I did so, however, people would give me a stunned look of horror and respond with,

"Oh no, you have got to get out of there."

"Who is *Bill?*" I would ask, only to be told that I would find out. And I did.

About a week later, the person I came to know as *Bill* came in. *Bill* turned out to be a short, bald, anemic-looking, chain-smoking man in a Hawaiian shirt, who looked like something that had just been dredged out of a river in a Hitchcock thriller. *Bill* was clearly *off-air* talent, with looks that deserved an "X" rating at that. *Bill* was not a nine to five man and appeared to come and go as he pleased – I later learnt this was because nobody would dare confront him about the issue. Far be it for me, then, to suggest that he observe the numerous *No Smoking* signs around the building.

Bill was the ultimate weapon in the war of attrition between engineers, artists and management. He was our nuclear warhead in the war of interfactional rivalry. I learnt that the engineers tolerated him, not only because he was good at what he did but, more importantly, because he was the last bastion between the engineering tribe and their inevitable descent into *artistic integrity* or *fiscal responsibility.*

When *Bill* first walked into our office – or should I say *Bill's Office* – he struck me as a man who was not distracted with minor pleasantries. His first action was to walk up to my desk, swipe his arm right across the top surface and throw all my possessions onto the floor. His greeting was both warm and sincere,

"Who the fuck are you and what are you fucking doing in my fucking office? What's this fucking shit doing on my fucking desk?"

Despite his prosaic entry, it was clear that *Bill* did not have Tourette Syndrome. I also soon realized that he hadn't thrown all my possessions on the floor and cursed me because he was angry or in a rage but, rather, because he was *Bill* - and that was just the way that *Bill* behaved. *Bill* was pure, primal engineer, unsullied by any of the niceties that make the rest of us engineers as sophisticated and erudite as we are.

Bill presented an entirely new language structure to me. Almost every sentence that emanated from his mouth contained either the words *fuck* or *shit* or any combinations thereof – sometimes as nouns, sometimes as verbs or adverbs or adjectives. Sometimes, even as phonetic punctuation, as in a typical *Bill* expression "Fuck Fuck Fuck" or "Shit Shit Shit".

Nothing that anyone had told me about *Bill* could have prepared me for his grand entrance, and I immediately developed acute *Easter Island Syndrome.* What was worse was the fact that, as the cloud of smoke wafted from the cigarette hanging from the side of his mouth, and into my face (still staring in stunned disbelief at his entrance), the realization dawned upon me that I was going to have to share an office with this guy for the next three months. And, as icing on the cake, they had asked him to supervise my project. Could this have been what Sister Kevin was referring to when she had warned me about those far away cows and their long horns?

My first reaction was that it was only for 12 weeks, which was really only 60 working days, and *Bill* came in at lunchtime and I went home at 5pm so, in total, we would only have to spend 1,080,000 seconds together. 1,080,000 seconds would pass in no time, and it wasn't that long, if you said it quickly enough. Of course I would also have to hold my breath for the entire 1,080,000 seconds in order to avoid passively ingesting his disgusting cigarette smoke – but then, how difficult could that be?

It wasn't just *Bill* that had obviously been sent by Sister Kevin as one of those far away cows with the long horns. Next door to *Bill's Office* was a studio where they recorded *voice over* work for the network. – particularly promotions for upcoming programs. On the days that they did recordings, there would be eight to ten continuous hours of voice-overs, filtering from the studio into *Bill's Office*. Sometimes, they would record a promotion over and over, and over and over again. After a day of listening to this symphony of monotonous background repetition, embellished with the foreground sound of *Bill's* expletives, and the constant haze of cigarette smoke, I could recite an entire week's program schedule for the network. To this day, I can still remember the entire evening program line up for New Year's Eve, 1980 which, I might add, has been of little value in day to day conversation since then. Perhaps it was this incessant repetition pounding into *Bill's* brain that had driven him to become what he was.

One week with *Bill* had passed and I had adapted the old prison calendar system by making a notch in my desk blotter for every day that I had had to endure with him. Only 990,000 seconds to go, I thought, and I would be free – not very long when you said it quickly. As I bade *Bill* farewell for the week, and he responded with his kindly,

"Just fuck off!"

it occurred to me that, having been at a television network for several weeks, I had not really seen much of the *on-air talent* or, indeed, anything that actually happened *on-air*. And, this didn't appear to be the sort of environment in which I particularly wanted to spend another 990,000 seconds with *Bill* and his expletive vocabulary – and, not being able to inhale for another 990,000 seconds was also becoming a serious issue. Maybe I should just quit.

As the thought of quitting crossed my mind, I finally fell upon my first *on-air talent* – Marmalade, the studio cat. Marmalade had made numerous appearances on children's programs and telethons organized by the network and, I figured, a celebrity was a celebrity even if the celebrity was a feline. I squatted down to pat Marmalade who, up to that point, had also been the friendliest and most refined employee of the network that I had encountered. As I patted Marmalade, however, I heard the sound of the most dulcet and refined voice come booming from above me.

"I see you've found my little friend."

For a few seconds, I assumed that Sister Kevin had organized for a direct audience with God. As it turned out, it wasn't quite God but the next best thing – the network's retired newsreader, who had been an icon from the 1950s up to his retirement in the late 1970s. Marmalade, it turned out, had been his own flesh and fur – a cat that had adopted the newsreader and managed his life for him, as cats are want to do.

After his on-air retirement, the endearing ex-newsreader had apparently been retained for public relations work with the network and, on this day, had been in search of his beloved feline. Sensing that I was not in the best of moods, he introduced himself and observed that he hadn't seen me at the network before. He also enquired about the project I was working on, and reflected on the fact that television studios could be rather cold and impersonal places. In the best of newsreader voices, he told me that if I ever felt lonely or frightened, that I should come and visit him in his office and he would make us tea. As he was about to walk off down the passageway, rather than saying goodbye, he gave me a very *news-readerly* sign-off,

"God Bless, and do have a wonderful weekend."

Our entire conversation lasted less than three minutes and, in that time, he had managed to elevate me from a mood of total despair to one of self-confidence. I never did need to take up the offer of tea, but his offer alone gave me sufficient resolve to stick to what I had been doing and the confidence to make the best of the remaining 990,000 seconds that I had to spend with *Bill* - which wasn't very long, especially if you said it quickly.

Almost two and a half decades had passed since that encounter and, so too, had the endearing newsreader that I had known in person for only a few minutes. I often wondered, since then, how much impact the things that we did and said, during the course of our lives, really had upon other people. For all of his thousands of news broadcasts, whenever I now think of that newsreader, I think of him not principally as a television personality, for there are many of those in the world, but as an uncommonly kindly man who, for no other reason than being a kindly man, appeared to have made a conscious decision to devote three minutes of his life to improving someone else's life. When he died, the death notices in the newspapers reflected the hundreds of other lives for whom he had done the same.

Ironically, *Bill* and I also eventually came to some form of mutual respect (friendship might be too strong a word) during our 1,080,000 seconds together. The most memorable *Bill-Episode* for me (and a rare triumph of engineering over art) occurred one evening when, an hour before the evening news was scheduled to go to air, the director managed to spill a cup of coffee into a vision mixer panel in the news studio's presentation control area. This was no ordinary director. In fact, he was the network's star television director who subsequently went on to direct a few internationally successful feature films and the international television feed for a worldwide sporting telecast. At that time, however, he clearly felt above his given station in life, and the spilled cup of coffee was *Bill's* excuse to bring him back down to earth. *Bill* was summoned to presentation control by the frantic director. Upon arriving, he glared at the director and then at the damaged vision mixer,

"Can't you fucking artistic people read fucking English?" *Bill* bellowed sarcastically, as he pulled the lit cigarette out of his mouth and pointed it towards the *No Food or Drink* sign that was prominently displayed, right next to one of the many *No Smoking* signs. The rather frazzled director was obviously too shaken to bring up the subject of *Bill's* cigarette and was more concerned about the evening news,

"Can you get it fixed in time?"

"No."

"Why not?"

Now, at this point, most engineers would have responded with technical details about what needed to be done – or perhaps even about the resources that were required. In any case, it was self evident that repairs would take a lot longer than an hour. But, *Bill* didn't use any of those responses. He chose the more upfront, direct reason,

"Because I fucking hate you, that's fucking why!"

And, with that, *Bill* stormed off back to his office, leaving the director with acute *Easter Island Syndrome*. The news had to go on without Bill's help and without vision mixing. And, with the news being a flagship program for a commercial network, it took all of two minutes viewing for the chief executive officer (CEO) to pick up the phone and call the director to find out what had gone wrong (or, more precisely, to tell him, in the most eloquent of business terms, why it should not have gone wrong).

I never thought for a moment that *Bill* had the time to hate anyone, nor was he angry about someone having spilled a cup of coffee, but what impressed me most was that it was his way of making it clear that he was to be treated with respect – all the time, not just when the occasion required a superficial facade of politeness.

The next morning, a highly contrite director walked into our office, ears still ringing from the CEO's admonishment, and politely asked whether *Bill* was in, and whether he had had a chance to attend to the vision mixer. I suggested that he come back later, when *Bill* deigned to come in, but the director suggested that I might just want to leave a little message for him, and to tell *Bill* that he was sorry about the coffee. Which I proudly did, not only on behalf of myself, but on behalf of all other engineers who seldom got the opportunity to witness such a spectacle.

I learnt a good many things in the 1,080,000 seconds that I worked with *Bill*, and these have remained with me during my career. For one thing, I learnt that there were people who were called gentlemen and that there were people who actually were gentlemen. The retired newsreader was a true gentleman and, in retrospect, I came to realize that so too was *Bill*. In the decades since then, I discovered, to my surprise, that there were many *Bills* in the world. Generally, they tended to alienate just about everyone around them because they didn't waste time with pleasantries, or by providing a *have a nice day* facade that was acceptable to the outside world. They were who they were, and what you saw was what you got.

When I looked back on my first job, I realized that, for all the *have a nice day* people that I encountered at the television network, none had actually gone to any great lengths to assist me. *Bill*, on the other hand, rough exterior and all, would spend hours and hours teaching me how to do things – when help was needed, *Bill* would help, and so I still look back fondly upon him.

There were profound side effects to having worked with *Bill*, however – the most significant being that one's vocabulary was seriously *Bill-ified* – to the extent that one was only fit for work on a barge canal, or as *off-air talent* on a television network. For example, if one went to a restaurant, then a typical order to a waiter would be along the following lines,

"I'll have the fucking carrot soup, followed by the fucking pasta primavera, and what's this fucking shit on the wine list?"

It was somewhat disconcerting to find that, after a Catholic upbringing and, up to that point in time, a total of 15 years of schooling and university, three months with *Bill* had caused the complete breakdown of speech patterns that had been developed over 20 years. And, the worst part of it was that one didn't realize that one was saying these things until people, who had never been *Bill-ified*, would stare back in the same stunned disbelief that I had had when I first met *Bill*. Clearly, I needed new role models.

By the mid 1980s, I had been working as a professional engineer for several years when the *Back to the Future* movies had arrived, thereby presenting another great scientific role model – the *Doc Emmet Brown* caricature of the mad scientist. His vocabulary was somewhat less descriptive than *Bill's* but at least he was a colorful icon for the next generation of scientific aspirants – complete with bulging eyes, wild white hair and a passion for science or, more specifically in his case, time travel. Ironically, the *Emmet Brown* caricature was extraordinarily like the very real physicist, Professor Julius Sumner Miller. Both characters were larger than life, even though one of them was real life. And, the message from both was that science and research were about passion, fun and adventure.

Several years after the vibrant *Doc Emmet Brown* caricature first appeared, the very real Professor Julius Sumner Miller passed away, in 1987. I can still remember clearly, to this day, the evening television news story of his final lecture in Australia, which he gave when terminally ill, and only a few weeks prior to his death in the United States. The cantankerous professor wiped the streaming tears from his tired, old eyes and bade farewell, for what he obviously knew to be the last time, to his students and to a country he had made a second home, with his *Jimmy-Cagneyesque* *"..And I thank you..."*. The attention subsequently turned to two of the students leaving the lecture, also in tears. When asked by a journalist what the lecture had meant to them and why they were upset, one of the teary-eyed teenage students simply replied,

"I think we have just witnessed the passing of a truly great man."

Julius Sumner Miller had devoted his entire life to inspiring the youth of the world, and the poignancy of two teenagers shedding tears at his farewell, and according a septuagenarian physicist the emotions that they would normally accord a teen pop star, was all the epitaph he required. The sad reality, however, was that there were very few, if any, real scientists to take the place of the Sumner Millers of the world and, were it not for the movie and television caricatures, the world of science would still be struggling for inspiring role models for young people. However, it was not until after I had been involved in research for some years that I discovered why this was the case.

If there was one thing that was evident to me after working as a professional engineer, it was that very few engineers (or scientists or accountants or economists – insert occupations here) actually had a passion for what they were doing. And, without role models who were passionate about what they did, the professional world quickly degenerated into a corporate career-climbing pattern – or, as they say the in the military, a *ticket-punching* exercise. Even in the scientific and research worlds, which were supposed to have a noble basis to them, the career climbers were everywhere.

I had always believed, on the other hand, that those who had been given the opportunity to have the levels of education that we had been fortunate enough to have, owed society more than the pursuit of a career, and had to develop a higher sense of purpose. These were my principles and (as Groucho Marx once said) if you don't like them, I have lots of others. In any case, I was sure that this quest for a higher sense of purpose also had a lot to do with Sister Kevin, her far away cows, and their long horns.

Now you might assume that the logical corollary to all of what I have been saying was for me to deliberately move into the world of science and research but, again, you would be entirely wrong. As it turned out, in my youthful exuberance, I had always assumed that, when applying for jobs, one always had to say "yes" to everything in order to get a job. When I was applying for a job with a production machinery manufacturer, one of the questions I was asked at an interview was whether I would be prepared to take a master's research degree with the job. Without having had any intention of doing a master's degree, of course I said "yes", on the assumption that this would soon be forgotten. Well, it wasn't forgotten and, several years later, I emerged with a Master of Engineering degree and ended up with another job managing research activities in a university research centre. I would be lying if I said that this was a difficult task in the early years, particularly because, at that time, the centre had no staff and no research students to manage. However, day by day, it grew to become something much larger.

No sooner had I completed the master's degree than I was asked whether or not I intended taking a PhD in engineering. Without having had any interest in doing a PhD, I again made the mistake of saying "yes", rather than arguing about the subject. With no intention of ever completing it when I commenced, I again found myself, several years later, holding on to a doctoral qualification in engineering.

The supreme sense of irony of this sequence of events has not escaped me to this day, particularly when I watch students struggling to achieve the sorts of qualifications that I always took for granted, and never viewed as any more than peripheral background noise to other day to day matters – I didn't even bother attending my own graduation ceremonies. I always looked upon my master's and PhD qualifications as being incidental and accidental, although my less charitable critics have referred to them more in terms of a travesty of the learning process.

In my mind, my almost-inadvertent completion of a master's degree and PhD confirmed my long held view that, in the final analysis, all our big decisions in life have already been made for us, and all that is left for us to do is to go along for the ride and make the best of the smaller ones. Our higher sense of purpose, therefore, needs to be based on making the best of what is handed to us at any given moment.

If this does not give you some sense of the *Twilight Zone*, then let me give you some more information which you may find of interest, and which will keep coming up during the course of this book. My doctoral research was in a relatively dry area of engineering (some would say, and have uncharitably said, downright boring) but the irony was that the outcomes accorded with my philosophy on life.

Basically, in engineering, we don't need a time machine to look into the future, because we can use computer simulation to extrapolate forward and get a sense of the future. In simple terms, my doctoral research was about how we make decisions when we use computers to control things, and about how far into the future we need to look in order to make good decisions about what we are doing now.

Superficially, one might assume that the further one looks into the future, the better one's current decisions will be. Interestingly, in my research, I discovered that, in an engineering control sense, a short glimpse into the future provided an improvement in decision making and, thereafter, the further one looked into the future, the decision making deteriorated. Why was this so? Basically, because the future, as it was predicted at one instant in time, seldom eventuated. Other events always intervened. Very much along the lines of life.

When I tried to explain my research to others, I always used a simple example. I would tell people to suppose that they were walking across a street to catch a bus and that, in the middle of the street, was a puddle. They had to make a decision as to whether to walk through the puddle or walk around it. They could take a short look into the future and say that if they walk around the puddle they will be dry, whereas if they walk through the puddle they will get wet. The best short-term decision is to avoid the puddle. However, if they try to look at the longer-term, then avoiding the puddle may delay their crossing and cause them to miss the bus. So, the best longer-term decision is to get wet and catch the bus.

The problem in complex engineering systems, as in life, is that the world is never that simple - in technical engineering terms, we refer to this phenomenon as *shit happens*. Going through the puddle may change the timing of the crossing, such that one gets run over by a passing car, thereby leaving the pedestrian wet, flattened and still missing the bus. So, in my doctorate, as in life, I always endeavored to make the best short-term choices and let the longer-term choices take care of themselves.

In reality, of course, a research doctorate, in any field, generally leads one to knowing almost everything about next to nothing, then parlaying that into a career in which one claims to know everything about everything, and eventually recognizing that one knows next to nothing about anything – at this point, one is generally appointed to the sorts of position I hold, where one manages entire research processes. People who have doctorates, and have worked in a research environment, will recognize the uncanny truth of my definition, even if they only admit it to themselves in the dark recesses of their own minds.

A good research doctorate does, however, give one an ability to readily decipher fact from fiction and opinion from fact. It also leads one to question everything (*Why is it so?*). When one goes to school, one assumes that books are all correct (because everything is in writing). One assumes that doctors are always correct, even when they prescribe things that cause a rapid deterioration in health:

"Just keep taking the blue pills and you'll be fine Mrs. Jones – make sure you only take the red pill if the blue ones turn out to be poisonous."

Prior to getting a doctorate, if one reads a movie review, or car review, or book review, then one assumes that the reviewer is an all-knowing expert about movies or cars or books. After one gets a doctorate, however, one never reads, or listens to, anything without asking (or at least thinking),

"What is your background to write or say this?" and *"What are the facts, as opposed to your personal opinions?"*

Whenever I act as an external examiner for doctoral theses from other universities, or whenever I meet people who have recently received their doctorates, they invariably tell me about the minutia of what they did in their research. What I always want to know is not what they did but what they learnt. Did they ask *why is it so?* Did they question their own outcomes? Did they develop a higher sense of purpose for what they were doing? Generally, I discovered that the answer was that people didn't, and their research tended to reflect that.

One of the reasons that this is the case is because education, in general, doesn't tend to instill a higher sense of purpose in students, and the entire process tends to degenerate into rote learning and coming up with the *right answer* – for which students are rewarded. This ends up manifesting itself even at the highest end of the education spectrum – the doctoral thesis. In order to remedy this, whenever I lectured to students, I always endeavored, in the first lecture, to convey to them the need to have this higher sense of purpose in learning and in life. To this end, I always psyched myself up for the first lecture by watching a video cocktail of *Goodbye Mr. Chips*, *To Sir With Love*, *Dead Poets Society* and *Mr. Holland's Opus*. With these for ammunition, I would deliver a 20 minute preliminary lecture which I always felt was both poignant and inspirational, only to be met with the traditional response:

"Will this be in the exam?"

"No."

"Then why are we doing it?"

Obviously, inspiring people to learn was proving to be more difficult than the movies made it appear. So much for poignant and inspirational lectures. Nobody ever asked Robert Donat, Sidney Poitier, Robin Williams or Richard Dreyfus "*Will this be in the exam?*" after they'd given their poignant and inspirational lectures. I guess that's what came from having a class that was full of paid extras or, perhaps, it was all just in the way they said it.

Notwithstanding the under-whelming response I was getting from teaching students, the postgraduate research side of things was going somewhat better. The little research centre, in which I had come to manage research activities (with no staff or students), had eventually grown to become a research institute with over a hundred doctoral candidates and nearly two hundred master's candidates to manage, and I was also the chair of institute's research committee. The task of managing had also grown considerably, but then so too had my organizational skills, and my work minimization and avoidance skills. Of the hundred doctoral candidates that I managed, 12 of these were my own research students.

In moving forward with this story, however, I need to intervene and explain to you how research in universities and research institutes operates. The first thing that you need to understand is that, for each area of research, there is an *international research community*. This *international research community* acts like a big international family – in much the same way as the Mafia, only without the loyalty or ethics. Those who have worked with academics will know only too well why this is so.

The problem is that research, unlike business, has not progressed culturally for hundreds of years. Even in business, people came to understand that there needed to be ongoing relationships between businesses and that these had to be based upon two parties both *winning* – whenever there was one winner and one loser, a relationship was damaged. When competitors were involved, the primary focus was not just on gaining a competitor's share but expanding the size of the cake – this was always viewed as a reasonable course of action because businesses were wealth creators. Researchers, however, always viewed themselves as wealth consumers and, if they ever got hold of a cake, as far as they were concerned, the size of the cake was fixed. If a competitor wanted a slice of cake, then that was one less slice that was available to the others.

On top of all of this, one had to superimpose the notion of *academic excellence* which, after all was said and done, was about being better than someone else – that is, winning. This was what I came to refer to as the *bigger idiot* theory of research – in academia, making someone else look dumber (i.e., a *bigger idiot*) was often viewed and rewarded as positively as actually being smarter. This was a phenomenon that had existed for hundreds of years in the world of research.

To make matters more complicated, the institute in which I worked was predominantly involved in collaborative industrial research. In some cases, research projects involved several universities and/or research institutes, combined with industry partners, all pretending to work together while actually fulfilling their own personal objectives. The incentive that was used to achieve this togetherness was typically a government funding program, and the end result of a collaboration was not unlike what one would expect from a group of alley cats squabbling over a mouse.

The task of managing these projects basically involved trying to tell each alley cat that, if they waited patiently, their mouse would grow and they could each have a larger piece. The mouse was usually a research student or postdoctoral researcher and, woe betide the mouse or project manager who tried to intervene between the alley cats during a feud.

I always told my research mice (students) that, if they succeeded in getting their doctoral qualifications in this environment, then their future was assured. And, surprisingly, more than twenty of my postgraduate research mice did survive the alley cats and pick up the refereeing skills necessary to complete their doctorates, and go on to bigger and better things, including metamorphosing into research alley cats in their own right.

Research alley cats are not unlike regular cats in the sense that they are very territorial – they spray their territory by writing research papers and try to prevent new research cats from entering. A new research cat, entering the territory of an old research cat, has to spray new research papers. The end result is a feud in which the two cats try to discredit each other's papers by tearing them to shreds, thereby leaving only the scent of the victorious cat's research papers behind for posterity.

You may think that this alley cat squabbling in research is a new or localized phenomenon – it is not. It was just the same in Italy for Galileo in the 17th Century; for John Harrison (the genius clockmaker) in Britain in the 18th Century, and for the Nobel prize winning physicists at the Princeton Institute in the United States in the early part of the 20th Century. And, very little has changed today – except that the feuds are presumably conducted by email.

Apart from being a feudal system, the other thing that one learns about research, after a very short space of time, is that it is very difficult to move from one area to another – a serious problem if someone gets bored with what they are doing. Each research community has its own language barrier to prevent alley cats from another neighborhood entering their alleyway. We engineers, for example, tend to speak in TLAs. For you non-engineers, TLAs are three letter acronyms. To make the move from one area to another even more difficult, one discovers that, even within branches of the same discipline, TLAs can mean different things. For example, in industrial engineering, an "FMS" is a flexible manufacturing system. In aerospace engineering, an "FMS" is a flight management system and, in electrical engineering, "FMS" refers to Ferro-magnetic-steel. In medicine, the language barrier to entry is the nomenclature that they use – descriptive words are composed of an absolute minimum of 27 syllables of concatenated Greek and Latin roots, despite the fact that less than 0.01 percent of the world's medical profession speaks either Greek or Latin.

At a more personal level, I can also tell you that, in the fiery debates that sometimes take place between medical researchers and engineering researchers, the medical researchers always claim to be doing *serious* research (as opposed to what they view as *non-serious*, or engineering-type research). *Serious* research, from a medical researcher's perspective, means donning a white laboratory coat and wearing a sour expression on one's face, presumably because the sour expression improves the quality and the *seriousness* of the research outcomes. Engineering researchers, on the other hand, don't generally take life as seriously as medical researchers take their *serious* medical research. So, quite often, even at a personal level, there are antipathies and barriers between the various research communities.

As if the language and personal barriers, arising from the research disciplines themselves, are not enough, governments around the world add to the problem by creating *research grant application forms*. These are forms that researchers have to complete in order to apply for money that can fund research. Being government-created forms, this also means that they are incomprehensible to those that have to complete them. So, in order to get research grants, one not only needs to be familiar with the language of one's specific field but also of the language of government.

Rather than give you an example of a *research grant application* form, which you may find too confusing, please allow me to demonstrate the difficulty of applying for funds by providing you with a much simpler example of the problem. Below, I have taken an extract from the *specific instructions* provided by the United States Internal Revenue Service (IRS) on how to fill in one of the boxes on their form (known as a W-8BEN form, revised January 2003):

> *"…If you are a disregarded entity with a single owner who is a foreign person and you are not claiming treaty benefits as a hybrid entity, this form should be completed and signed by your foreign single owner. If the account to which a payment is made or credited is in the name of the disregarded entity, the foreign single owner should inform the withholding agent of this fact. This may be done by including the name and account number of the disregarded entity on line 8 (reference number) of the form. However, if you are a disregarded entity that is claiming treaty benefits as a hybrid entity, this form should be completed and signed by you."*

Can anyone guess what question these specific instructions are designed to assist one in answering? These instructions – I kid you not – were designed to help a person to fill out the box marked *Name* on an IRS form. Now, if one multiplies the complexity of these helpful instructions by a factor of ten, for research grant application forms, then one has some insight into why a PhD is required to get government research resources – it has little to do with the research and much to do with how difficult it is to fill out the forms.

The other fascinating thing that one discovers about research grant application forms is that the people who generate them have never actually filled them in – the end result being that a text box for *telephone number* is half a page in size, whereas the text box left for *summarize the project in 300 words* is smaller than an Ethiopian postage stamp.

The *Professor* on *Gilligan's Island*, *Dr Smith* on *Lost in Space, and Doc Emmet Brown* in *Back to the Future*, all had, by television or movie voodoo, an unlimited supply of resources and an ability to do whatever they pleased – even if, in the case of *Gilligan's Island*, these resources only amounted to coconuts. For real researchers, in a world of limited resources, there are initiation rites to getting those resources, particularly from government. One of these is to have credentials based on research papers that have been reviewed by peers and published in international journals. This is a way of ensuring that a researcher is serious about a field before receiving access to resources.

In the early part of the 20th Century, even the most notable researchers, in the then burgeoning area of physics, may have published only one or two dozen significant research papers in an entire lifetime. This made sense because each significant research paper would have required several years of research. By the end of the 20th Century, the global trend towards measuring research outcomes (by publications and citations) meant that all researchers had, magically, boosted their publications to the stage where every quack university professor on the planet would lay claim to having authored hundreds of research papers. Since it wasn't possible to achieve such an outcome in any legitimate research sense, it was justified by claiming that papers had been co-authored with research students and underlings – hence that the publications were an accurate reflection of the ability to generate research funding.

With this formula of *more is better* in mind, one now needs to understand that research has also become a big, big business. At a global level it is a multi-billion dollar business and a major employer. Government, military, university and benefactorial research institutions around the world collectively employ hundreds of thousands of staff and research students. And, for all the research marketing hyperbolae about the betterment of mankind, no-one is likely, in the near future, to stand up and say,

"Can you believe it, we've just found a generic cure for the XYZ disease – just eat a banana and a bag of peanuts every day for a week – how could we have missed that? Now we can shut down all these incredibly costly research institutes, put thousands of researchers out of work and spend the money on something more worthwhile,"

and be thanked for it by the research community.

Yet, that is what the public perceives to be going on in the *cloud cuckoo-*

land of the research world – clear cut goals with a tangible end point. This is the public's big picture, or the *champagne for tomorrow* scenario which is applied by research spin-doctors to raise money. The picture from a researcher's perspective is a lot smaller, and operates on the *glass of water for today* scenario. Researchers view the world as an ongoing series of grant applications, which are used to fund research that leads to research papers, which leave many unanswered questions, and lead to more grant applications to fund more research, to lead to more research papers, that lead to more unanswered questions that require more funding. In other words, a self sustaining industry. There is no Machiavellian intent behind this philosophy, it is just the way that things are because there is nothing to break the cycle of the research merry-go-round.

As wars are said to cause *collateral damage*, so too, one learns that research sometimes ends up causing *collateral outcomes*. That is, things which are of benefit to society or industry, despite the best efforts of researchers and government granting bodies to keep the merry-go-round running. However, turning this research merry-go-round into a consistent production line for outputs is a difficult task.

In the 18th Century, the British Government recognized this problem of the research merry-go-round and endeavored to put a stop to it by announcing an enormous financial reward for anyone solving an important research problem – measuring longitude at sea. The end result was that they were flooded with thousands of crackpots and charlatans endeavoring to claim the prize, and a judging panel that was open to (and accused of) bias and corruption. So, while all those who ride the research merry-go-round recognize that it does not have an *off switch*, there have been very few viable alternatives put forward.

You also need to understand that this is where industry-funded, applied research and fundamental (or basic or pure) research differ. When industry funds applied research, it pays for measurable, clear-cut outcomes on finite time-lines. Fortunately, for the researchers, industrial research is self sustaining because technology is constantly evolving and markets are constantly changing. However, in some areas of fundamental research, such as medicine, the big research areas have a definite end point. Anyone who enters the arena with the *banana and bag of peanuts* solution immediately pulls the power plug out of the socket for the merry-go-round. Human nature being what it is, one knows that this is not likely to happen.

Armed with this knowledge, I always encouraged my research students to make sure that they followed and understood the money-trail before they looked at the research-trail, for the money-trail creates reasons in research that reason itself does not know. In research, the money trail can generally be traced by asking five basic questions:

- *Who funds the research?*

- *Who sits on the committees that decide where the money is spent?*

- *Who gets the money that the committees allocate?*

- *Who are the beneficiaries of the research outcomes?*

- *Which research outcomes provide the greatest financial benefits?*

In industrial research, the money-trail is relatively straightforward – industry puts money in to get tangible products or intellectual property (IP) or services out – which they intend to sell in some way. For all the academic fears of participating in industry research, it is unusual to find an instance where industry perverts the actual course of applied research – primarily because they are predominantly interested in commercial outcomes and things that actually work. My experience was that, generally, there were considerable benefits in having industry fund applied research and relatively few problems. The big problems, however, arose when industry funded fundamental research, such as in the medical arena.

In medical research, the money-trail is quite complicated and the stakes are often extraordinarily high. Pharmaceutical companies often sponsor fundamental medical research. This, in itself, can cause major ethical dilemmas for participants. For one thing, pharmaceutical companies haven't traditionally made money from healthy people, and they don't make sufficient money from *silver bullet* cures (where a single pill, taken once, cures an ailment) to amortize the enormous costs associated with drug research, testing, development and commercialization.

Cash flow in the pharmaceutical world is sustained by selling products that have to be taken for long periods of time, preferably indefinitely. The cash cows of the pharmaceutical world include drugs such as those for hypertension, depression, diabetes, PD, Multiple Sclerosis, etc. And, if medical research shows that dosages need to be increased, or that the thresholds at which medication starts need to be lowered, then the changes to the bottom lines of pharmaceutical companies can often be measured in billions of dollars.

More recently, the pharmaceutical world also recognized that there were billions more dollars to be made by getting healthy people to take *just-in-case* drugs on a permanent basis. These are the sorts of drugs that the pharmaceutical world would like people to take when they are healthy, so that they are (theoretically) less likely to get sick later. After all, why should healthy people be excused from buying pharmaceutical products just because they don't actually need them? To this end, medical research programs are funded to prove that healthy people who take *just in case* drugs are less likely to get sick than those who don't. Such research programs are akin to having people spray themselves with alligator-repellent, and then discovering that 99.99% of all people who use alligator-repellent never get eaten by alligators. Fortunately for the pharmaceutical companies who fund such programs, research that proves such a hypothesis also has the potential to add billions of dollars to the bottom line.

The scale of the financial benefits of such research programs can therefore be immense, depending on the outcomes. Moreover, given the stakes, the very nature of research programs can be skewed to achieve those outcomes. For example, it is unusual to have research studies undertaken on the positive health benefits of decreasing pharmaceutical usage, because obviously this is of little interest to those who fund such programs, or influence government policy on what gets funded.

At the core of all these ethical problems (and, perhaps, exacerbating them) is the tendency for educational systems to try and breed people, particularly researchers, to go in search of the *right* answer and never actually question the systems that are in place. As you go through this book, you may begin to realize why these issues are particularly important in areas such as medical research. Fortunately, however, unlike medical researchers, an engineer, such as myself, never had to deal with ethical issues of this magnitude.

The other important factor which differentiates we engineering researchers from our medical research counterparts is that human beings aren't all manufactured to the same exacting tolerances. When God said, "*Let there be light*", we engineers already had the wiring in place, and have worked hard to maintain reliability, consistency and quality in the world ever since. If only God had taken as much care in manufacturing humans as we engineers took in manufacturing *Toyotas*, then medical research would be considerably easier. Trends and correlations in engineering tend to be much stronger, and can more readily be validated because we deal with identical systems and have rigorous controls. It is much more difficult for our medical counterparts to find genetically identical humans with which to conduct their experiments and, so, trends tend to be less clear cut and the variations from sample to sample are often significant.

In science and engineering, it is simply not sufficient to say that a correlation exists between one phenomenon and another – there needs to be determined a physical relationship that demonstrates why a correlation exists – why is it so? Correlations can exist between two phenomena for a range of reasons. For example, if one takes ten people who wear hats, and cuts off their ears, then there might be a very strong correlation between cutting off ears and blindness – is this because cutting off ears causes blindness, or because cutting off ears causes people's hats to fall down over their eyes? There might also be a high correlation between people eating cabbages, 24 hours a day, and not getting lung cancer – is this because of something in the cabbages or because people are so busy eating cabbages that they don't have time to smoke? This is where the role of good scientists and engineers gets a lot tougher.

In medical research, correlations are plentiful – the difficulty is that the physiological and biochemical theories that bind one phenomenon to another are so complex and multidimensional that determining whether or not a correlation is meaningful is often difficult or intractable. Moreover, the propensity for vested interest groups to make use of correlations in medical research, in the absence of physical linkages, is significantly higher than in engineering. Hence, my developed philosophy, of always focusing on the money-trail before looking at the research-trail, is especially useful when examining medical research claims.

The *Professor* on *Gilligan's Island* never seemed to have to tackle the issues of research ethics, or multinational pharmaceutical companies, or other vested interest groups, when making radio batteries out of coconut shells. *Doc Emmet Brown* didn't have to get ethics approval for experimenting on humans and dogs in his time machines. Thankfully, for most of my research life, neither did I. However, I did regularly come across this problem of correlating one phenomenon to another and working out whether the correlation was meaningful.

One case in point was where we had a doctoral research student looking at the quality of spot welds produced by robots in the car industry. Ordinarily, quality was assessed by destructive testing of a sample of welds. Destructive testing is little more sophisticated than testing matches to see if they work by lighting them – once they've been tested it doesn't much matter whether they worked or not. Our objective was to see if a more sophisticated approach could be developed. The end result of the project was a system that monitored the acoustic emissions (sounds) produced when a weld occurred. A *good* weld had a unique sound signature. Each type of *bad* weld also had its own unique sound signature. By looking at the sound signatures, one could automatically determine whether or not a defective weld had occurred. Of course, while the correlations were clear, there also had to be determined a scientific basis for why the sounds of welds varied according to the quality of the weld.

The moral of this spot-welding story is that, in engineering, we cannot always measure what we want so, instead, we measure what we can, and then see whether or not this can be meaningfully correlated to what we want. In medicine, however, the emphasis is predominantly on measuring what we want – that is, physically analyzing a blood sample or getting an image of a region of the body. This is not always straightforward and one might assume that medicine could also benefit from investigating some of the engineering techniques that are in common usage – measure what you can and correlate it to what you want – the hard part, of course, is determining whether a correlation is meaningful.

My interest in applying engineering principles to medicine was only by way of passing curiosity until, one day, as chair of our institute's research committee, it was brought to my attention that our institute had a doctoral research student who was undertaking research into just such an area. The objective of the student's research was to develop a computer control system for a neo-nate crib for premature infants. The idea was to control the climate of the crib while monitoring an infant's *core* body temperature. The *core* body temperature is one indicator of potential problems, such as viral or bacterial infections – it is not the same as the surface temperature, which varies with exercise, etc.

The problem with getting *on-line core* body temperature measurements, which can be fed into a computer system, is that temperature is a difficult parameter to accurately measure using non-invasive devices. The more accurate (invasive), traditional thermometers provided potential sources of discomfort and infection for neo-nates. The student's task was therefore to develop an accurate, non-invasive system that could be incorporated into the computer control system for a crib.

For a number of reasons, it was decided that it would be difficult for the candidate to get ethical approval to do any meaningful testing and it was also decided that, as chair of the research committee, I should take over the supervision of the candidate and find a new focus for the project. In the research world, people are hesitant about inheriting students because each supervisor has their own style of supervision, and that means that an inherited student often comes with the baggage of the previous supervisor, which sometimes causes conflicts. My initial reaction was therefore no. However, it was subsequently explained to me that there were three options. Specifically that:

(i)   As chair of the institute's research committee, I should feel guilty and that I should take the research student

(ii)   I should "stop my bitching and moaning" and just take the research student

(iii)   Since there was no-one else within our institute or university who would take the student mid stream, and our institute had a formal commitment, and I was the chair of the research committee, then I should take the research student.

Not being one to respond to ultimata, I was at least pleased that these three options had been presented, and I decided to take the research student.

The first thing that had to be done was to review what the research student had been doing and, given the ethics situation, determine what new focus the research project should have. This, I did, by asking him to come and meet with me and submit his existing literature review. I discovered that my new charge was still brimming with enthusiasm and passion for what he was doing. Shouldn't take more than a few months to drag him down into the gutter and have him at the same level of deadpan cynicism that I have, I thought.

Upon reading the literature review, I discovered that the research student had been looking at earlier research which showed that, interestingly, the core body temperature of humans could be indirectly measured by observing the brain's response to auditory signals (sounds) – this was the so-called auditory brainstem response, or ABR (also known as the auditory evoked brainstem response or AEBR).

Now, as an engineer, the sum total of my knowledge of the human brain, up until that point in time, was that it was located somewhere above the feet and somewhere below the hat – if one wore a hat. The only other piece of knowledge I had about brains was that, if one went to fancy restaurants, they sometimes appeared on exotic menus disguised under the euphemism of *sweetbread* – never order the *sweetbread*, was my only other piece of knowledge about brains. Nevertheless, even with this meager knowledge it still occurred to me to ask the obvious question of, why is it so? Why should an individual's core body temperature correlate with the brain's response to sounds? The answer, I discovered, from reading the literature review, was that the brain ultimately controlled the body's thermoregulatory system and, hence, there was published research relating the performance of the brain to the core temperature of the body.

This correlation between core body temperature and auditory brain response was all well and good but it appeared that this research had already been done some time ago. What were we supposed to do now?

To resolve this problem I turned to my think tank, which is not a group of highly intelligent people but, rather, a tank (swimming pool) in which I think. Every morning, before starting work, I swim 3500 meters, which is 70 laps of a 50 meter pool. Now, if you are a goldfish, and have a memory span of less than 15 seconds, then this is not a problem because every time you bump into a wall to do a flip turn, it seems like a new wall and you feel as though you have just had a new life experience. However, if you are like me and have a memory span of several minutes, or more, then bumping into the same walls, 70 times, can become rather dull (you will recall I have already touched upon the subject of engineers being rather dull). To remedy this, I traditionally spend the upward laps convincing myself that I am an Olympic swimming champion, and the downward laps thinking about what I am going to be doing at work. A swimming pool is a good place to do undisturbed thinking because there are no telephones or unexpected visitors. And, as long as one remembers to flip-turn every 50 meters, concussion from bumping into the end walls can generally be minimized.

The subject of what to do with this new research student consumed some 17,500 meters of pool thought (which is how I measure my brain activity in the pool) over a couple of weeks. The obvious course of action to remedy the ethics problems was to move away from infants to consenting adults but then, what was the point of having this elaborate technique for measuring core body temperature on adults when one could just use a regular thermometer?

Somewhere around the 5,000 meter thought mark, it occurred to me that the auditory brainstem response was presumably an indicator of other neurological phenomena as well as core body temperature. Presumably, it was already used for some diagnostic purposes apart from hearing tests. By the 7,000 meter thought mark, I had convinced myself that the research student should investigate both the current and potential uses of ABR for diagnostic purposes – but, to what end?

Some months earlier, a television documentary had been screened on the claims that the discredited 1960s pharmaceutical drug, *Ecstasy* (which subsequently became an illegal substance or, euphemistically, a *recreational* drug), had shown a rapid improvement in the condition of one PD victim in Britain. In the documentary, they screened *before and after* videos of the patient, who alleged that there had been some improvement as a result of taking the (by then) illegal substance. Leaving aside the obvious problem of a sample size of one, when I had discussed this with a colleague, who was a hospital-based medical specialist, he responded with some skepticism and the obvious question of how they knew that the person had PD in the first place.

I was informed, to my surprise, that they did not currently have a definitive diagnostic tool for the disease other than autopsy, which wasn't particularly useful to those who were still breathing and enduring the disease. So, any assessment of whether or not the person on the documentary was a genuine patient was really a matter of educated guesswork for an experienced clinician. I subsequently learnt that a specialized form of medical imaging, referred to as *flourodeoxyglucose-based positron emission tomography* (fPET) scanning had been used, for some time, to detect the presence of the disease. However, fPET was a high cost method of doing medical imaging and was unsuited for use as an on-line tool that could be applied by practitioners, on a regular basis, to monitor changes that occurred or, indeed, the progression of the disease.

By the 8,000 meter thought mark, the other thing that had crossed my mind – putting all these unsubstantiated pieces of rubbish together – was that I had read somewhere that a number of young-onset Parkinson's patients had first sought medical attention because they had experienced some form of thermal overload while jogging or playing sport. At the 9,000 meter thought mark, I had managed to convince myself, with little more than unsubstantiated, garbled, second-hand knowledge of a field, about which I knew absolutely nothing, that the research student should determine whether auditory brain response could be used as a diagnostic tool for PD. In other words, did people with Parkinson's have a different ABR to people without?

Approaching the 10,000 meter thought mark, I reflected on what must have surely existed in regard to knowledge about the disease. At a micro (or molecular) level, I thought to myself, the pharmaceutical companies must have already performed some form of detailed modeling of the performance of Parkinson's medication. After all, this represented a whole field of science called pharmacokinetics – this must have already been well established after so many years, I assumed. But, at a macro level, where they needed to have detailed knowledge of how a patient's overall condition changed with medication – how could they, if they weren't even able to readily diagnose the disease in the first place?

At the 11,000 meter thought mark, I already had visions of a Nobel Prize firmly in hand, and thanking all those *little* people who had helped – too numerous to mention by name but, *"they know who they are"*. But why stop at just one Nobel Prize, while I was on a roll? The other thing that I had seen on PD, on a US current affairs program, was about the idiosyncrasies of the medication. It had remained in my memory only because of the unintentional, Vaudevillian faux pas in the narrative, along the lines of,

"...an hour after taking the drug Sinemet, 'X' was able to play the piano..."

This had led those engineers among us, who were watching, to comment on what a tremendous drug this *Sinemet* must be. Could different drugs enable us to play different types of musical instruments? Could we, for example, play the banjo several hours after taking an antibiotic or, perhaps, the cello after taking an antihistamine?

If the analysis of an auditory brain response signature correlated with the presence of PD, then the simplicity of such a monitoring process also meant that one could log the effects of medication on brain response over, say, 24 hours, and potentially provide insights into better medication regulation and quality of life. Even if the dissipation rate of the medication in the body had been modeled by the pharmaceutical companies in their pharmacokinetic studies, its macro impact upon the brain response may not necessarily be known. If one could monitor the actual impact of the medication by using a measurable quantity (rather than clinical observation), then one could more accurately map out the effect of the medication, as a function of time.

More disturbingly, however, a number of research papers had revealed that the misdiagnosis rate of PD was estimated by some researchers at up to 25% of those presenting to neurologists with clinical symptoms – this was a figure prominently quoted by medical imaging companies in the United States. However, given that these companies derived a healthy income from lauding the misdiagnoses of neurologists, this number probably represented an upper extreme. Neurologists, on the other hand, reported that the more recent figure was a lot better, at under 5%, due to better training of clinicians. The neurologists, of course, derived a healthy income from convincing patients that they had the expertise to diagnose and manage the disease, and so this number probably represented a lower extreme. Applying the wisdom of Solomon (who probably knew as much about PD as I did) to these numbers, I surmised that the figure was probably in the order of 10%, which was still significant.

This, of itself, would have been of concern but, worse still, was the fact that after an initial clinical diagnosis, a second stage, makeshift test for the disease involved prescribing Parkinson's medication and assessing its impact – the greater the impact of the medication, the more likely one was to conclude a patient actually had the disease. The numbers were quite staggering when one considered that around one in every two hundred people in some (ageing) societies were diagnosed with the disease. And, in the worst case scenario, one quarter of those was unnecessarily receiving Parkinson's medication.

It wasn't just that a misdiagnosis inflicted undue stress upon those who did not have the disorder – the recipients of the second phase test were also exposed to all the side effects of the medication as well – and these were highly unpleasant to say the least.

At the 12,000 meter mark, my thoughts turned to the money trail and the notion that PD was really God's gift to the pharmaceutical world. Could anyone possibly conceive, in their wildest imagination, in any area of endeavor, of a better business? One in every two hundred people was forced to indefinitely purchase a product which treated symptoms but didn't actually cure the problem for which it was developed – even then, there were severe side effects – and, those got worse the longer one used the product.

Many of the users of Parkinson's medication would never think of complaining about the product because their neurologists often presented the product to them as *"not a cure; not 100% effective at alleviating the symptoms, and full of side effects – don't worry if you feel nauseous, dizzy, constipated and have hallucinations – that's perfectly normal"*. And, as icing on the cake, around a tenth of the product sales were to people who probably didn't need to be taking it in the first place.

At the 12,500 meter mark, I was doing the arithmetic. If, say, two out of the five billion people in the world had sufficient wealth to buy pharmaceuticals then, at any point in time, there were around ten million *life-long* customers for PD medication. The Mayo Clinic had estimated the pharmaceutical market for PD to be worth six billion dollars per year in the US alone. And somewhere around one million people in the worldwide customer base were presumably purchasing the product (for an average of several months) because they had been misdiagnosed. Misdiagnosis was as good, financially, for the pharmaceutical world, as selling an additional million television sets a year was for the electronics industries. Clearly, from a business perspective, any silver bullet cure for the disorder would have big repercussions. But then, even a definitive diagnostic tool for PD would put a sizeable dent into the bottom line of pharmaceutical sales.

By the 13,000 meter thought mark, however, my impending Nobel Prize had slipped from my grasp, and so too had all the *little* people, too numerous to mention. Pursuing this line of research would be pointless. Back to the realities - this would be an *orphan* project that would take place without the imprimatur of a recognized research institute in the field; with an engineer endeavoring to get ethics clearance past medical people in order to conduct tests on patients; with patients who would have to trust an engineer, and by liaising with neurologists who, in all probability, would not give us the time of day, much less thank us for wasting their time with *"don't you think it would be a good idea if..."*

On top of all of these problems was the *none too minor* issue that I didn't really know the first thing about medicine, biology, biochemistry, the neurosciences, human experimentation, clinical testing or, for that matter, basic human research ethics. I wasn't likely to develop a lifetime's worth of professional expertise in the field over a couple of years of peripheral reading. So, even if we did end up finding a correlation between the auditory brainstem response and some Parkinson's related phenomenon, we wouldn't have the knowledge that would be required to put forward any remotely plausible physiological basis for it. That would leave the whole research exercise ending with gaping holes in it. I could already envision the thesis examiners' comments:

"Well no wonder they got these ridiculous results – they did the experiments on a Tuesday – that always happens when you measure auditory brainstem response on a Tuesday..."

That is the fundamental problem with meddling in a research area in which you have no core professional expertise. Added to these obstacles, of course, was the minor detail that my entire understanding of the human brain was that it was located somewhere above the feet and somewhere below the hat. What if Parkinson's patients didn't wear hats?

On top of which, it finally dawned upon me that I was now responsible for the outcomes of a doctoral research program in the area, and that the research student, if unable to reach an international standard in his research, will have wasted three years of his life and will have me, as his principal supervisor, to thank for it. I figured that if I stopped swimming at the pool, and just started swimming in the Pacific Ocean instead, after three years I might be sufficiently far out of his reach to avoid his wrath.

Coming up to the 17,000 meter thought mark, I asked myself what would the greats do? Did the *Professor's* lack of batteries, on *Gilligan's Island,* prevent him from making some out of coconut shells? Of course not. Did the fact that there was no such thing as Inter-galactic Space Science prevent *Dr. Zachary Smith* from getting a PhD in the field in *Lost in Space*? Of course not. Did the fact that the *flux-capacitor* was a cheap screenwriter's ruse, with no basis in engineering, prevent *Doc Emmet Brown* from using it for time travel in *Back to the Future*? Of course not. And what would Julius Sumner Miller have done? He had died of course – an omen perhaps?

At the 17,250 meter mark, I asked myself how difficult could this be? After all, am I not an engineer? And, isn't an entire medical degree little more than an instruction manual and road map for the human body? And, do we engineers need or read instruction manuals or road maps? Of course not. We could make the transition to *serious* research. All that would be required was a white laboratory coat and a sour expression on one's face.

By the 17,500 meter mark, I decided that things were going ahead, and that was that. In the back of my mind, however, I still had doubts, and visions started to emerge of the *off-ramp* from the *engineering freeway* leading to that cornball and fabled *road less travelled* – and this wasn't an *off-ramp* I had planned to take.

Nevertheless, I thought, whether or not any correlations could be found with this ABR stuff, there was sufficient work for the student to get a doctoral qualification. I therefore asked my new research student to see if he could find a second supervisor for the project, with whom he was comfortable, and he said that he would. I organized the first formal meeting with the student and the new co-supervisor, whom I understood was also an electrical engineer, and began my preparatory work.

After desperately downloading everything that I could find on PD from the Internet, I decided that the best way to assert my authority on the project was to impress both the student and the other supervisor with my vast knowledge of the subject. Desperate times called for desperate measures - memorization and rote learning would be required – morals would have to be checked in at the door. And, if all else failed, no-one could help but be impressed with my detailed understanding of the brain – located somewhere above the feet and somewhere below the hat.

As I waited for the others to arrive at my office for the first meeting, I gave myself a final,

"*...Well Toto, looks like we're not in Kansas anymore...*"

and then welcomed them in. The landing in *Munchkin-land*, however, proved to be somewhat rougher than I had anticipated.

I started the meeting with my crude, rote-learnt presentation on PD, which I was graciously allowed to continue for about fifteen minutes.

I explained the basics of the disease, including the fact that it was caused by the depletion (death) of a particular group of neurons in the brain. These neurons had the task of producing a chemical known as Dopamine, which was one of a group of *neurotransmitters*. The role of the Dopamine was to facilitate the transmission of signals from the brain to various muscles. The lack of Dopamine production led to sporadic problems in the transmission of these signals, and hence a broad range of movement disorders. I also explained the actions of the various medications, used to replicate the production of Dopamine in the brain, and their side effects.

I could have gone on longer and explained about my personal knowledge of the brain, and how it was located somewhere above the feet and below the hat. However, as fate would have it, in the midst of my rote-learnt explanation, I finally succumbed to my ignorance of the subject; stumbled on an expression and paused.

"You mean the blood-brain barrier?" queried the new co-supervisor.

"Yes, that's the expression I'm looking for," I replied. And, then came my fateful question, which I should have asked up front,

"What did you say your area of expertise was?"

"Well, my background is in psychophysiology and, for the last ten years, I've been working in the sensory neurosciences area."

As I slowly felt myself dissolving into my chair in embarrassment, I knew, for the first time, how Margaret Hamilton had felt in the *Wizard of Oz* as she melted into the ground. There was just no point in overwhelming this guy with my knowledge of the brain being located somewhere above the feet and somewhere below the hat – they probably taught that in psychophysiology school or wherever the hell he went to get his PhD.

"Do you have one of those neat plastic brains in your office?" I enquired, still rather red faced.

"Yes, actually I do," he responded.

"Alright then."

It was an inauspicious beginning. Fate had led us to tackle a project which would require us to acquire a brain, heart and courage – at least we already had a brain, albeit a plastic one. Although the project required heart, after all I've told you about engineers, you should know by now that we engineers don't use or require hearts, and if you ever send an engineer out in search of one, they will only return with a multi-point fuel injection system instead. That only left the courage that would be required to pick up the phone and start calling the various PD organizations to ask for their support in getting participants.

"And what did you say your area of specialization was again doctor?" They will ask.

"...Actually, I'm an engineer...Hello...Hello...have we been cut off? Is anybody still out there?"

2 OF BARTLEBY AND PARKINSON'S DISEASE

"Ah Bartleby. Ah humanity."

So ended, in melodramatic style, Herman Melville's 1853 story, *Bartleby the Scrivener – a Story of Wall Street*. Although Melville was more renowned for his book *Moby Dick*, scholars are far more infatuated with *Bartleby*, and I will endeavor to explain to you why I think *Bartleby* and his story are of importance here too.

I think that it is only fair to tell you that *Bartleby* and Melville are not things which are normally discussed in the inner sanctum of the most secret of engineering societies. Many engineers have difficulty differentiating between Dylan Thomas and Bob Dylan; George Bernard Shaw and George Burns – and, for that matter, Walt Whitman and Walt Disney. For this reason, engineers generally wait for classic literature to come out on DVD, in mini-series format, so that it can be appreciated in the manner in which engineers believe that authors, such as Shakespeare, would have intended – in fast forward, and skipping over the scenes which they feel are unnecessary.

At this point, however, I need to differentiate myself from some of my engineering counterparts and tell you that I do read (and write) significantly more than they generally do, as a result of the various positions that I have held. And, of the many hundreds of books I have read, one that has always stood out is the story of *Bartleby*, because it is a simple parable with very complex connotations. For those who haven't read the work, I will endeavor not to diminish it but, rather, to merely summarize it and its implications.

To begin with, it needs to be explained that a scrivener, as the name suggests, was a writer or, more precisely, a human photocopier. In Melville's book, *Bartleby*'s story is set in a legal firm, which operates in New York's Wall Street in the 19th Century, and which derives an income from doing work on mortgages, bonds and legal deeds – hence the need for human photocopiers.

The man who relates the story of *Bartleby* is the unnamed, elderly owner of the legal firm, who introduces himself with his proud conviction that *"the easiest way of life is the best"*. He also introduces us to two of his employees, who have been given the nicknames of *Turkey* and *Nippers*. *Turkey* is a man who, in the prosaic words of Melville, *"prosperity harmed"*. *Turkey*'s capacities appear to be seriously diminished after lunch, presumably due to the demon drink. *Nippers*, on the other hand, is described as a man for whom *"nature herself seemed to have been his vintner"*. Although *Nippers* does not drink, his personality and indigestion diminish his capacity prior to lunch. However, the owner of the firm is prepared to tolerate both *Turkey*'s and *Nippers*' flaws and eccentricities because, in his words, *"their fits relieved each other like guards."* And, in the final analysis, he surmises that *"Nippers, like his compatriot Turkey, was a very useful man to me."*

The arrival of *Bartleby*, the new scrivener, is initially a source of great satisfaction and pride to the owner because he appears to have no flaws, and a passion for the tedious and dehumanizing work of copying documents by hand:

> *"I cannot credit that the mettlesome poet Byron would have contentedly sat down with Bartleby to examine a law document of, say, five hundred pages, closely written in a crimpy hand."*

On his third day at work, however, when the owner asks *Bartleby* to perform a simple task, *Bartleby* responds with *"I would prefer not to"* – which becomes his defiant catch-cry throughout the book. The owner of the legal firm is both startled and furious at such defiance. And, no amount of pleading or threatening is able to change *Bartleby*'s mind:

> *"…nothing so aggravates an earnest person as a passive resistance."*

Unable to manage *Bartleby*'s defiance, and unable to bring himself to dismiss the scrivener, the owner decides to just tolerate him. However, after some 32 days, the owner discovers that *Bartleby* has moved into the legal chambers to live, apparently because he has no place else to go. The owner also discovers that all the copying that *Bartleby* has performed, by candlelight, has damaged his eyes. *Bartleby* has therefore decided to give up his copying, but will not leave the owner's employ. Eventually, the owner decides to ask him to leave and offers to assist with his relocation – but *Bartleby* does not leave because he *"prefers not to…"*

Exasperated, but still retaining some compassion, the owner decides to move to new offices, rather than to confront *Bartleby* again. Although *Bartleby* is locked out of the new offices, the owner is paid a visit by another lawyer who tells him that *Bartleby* has still not left the old chambers. As a gesture of goodwill, the owner decides to return to his old offices to try and persuade *Bartleby* to move, which he refuses to do, because *Bartleby* *"would prefer not to."* Completely exasperated, the owner feels that he can do no more and leaves *Bartleby* to his fate, which is to be taken and locked away in the *Tombs* of New York.

Filled with remorse, the owner eventually decides to visit the imprisoned *Bartleby* to assuage his own guilt:

"…it was not I who brought you here, Bartleby."

With a pang of compassion, he slips some silver into the prison *grub-man's* hands, so that he may feed *Bartleby* more generously. However, having been removed from his office home and imprisoned, *Bartleby* has become depressed and moribund – *Bartleby* *prefers not to* eat. The owner cannot understand *Bartleby's* depression:

"…And to you, this should not be so vile a place. Nothing attaches to you by being here. And see, it is not so sad a place as one might think. Look, there is the sky, and here is the grass."

Bartleby, however, continues to refuse meals and wastes away, only for the owner to eventually find him on a subsequent visit – huddled at the base of a stone wall in the *Tombs*, asleep with – in Melville's words – *kings and counselors.*

The owner's final, enigmatic cry of *"Ah Bartleby. Ah humanity."* has been debated by scholars for more than one and a half centuries. Was it Melville's parody on the melodramatic endings of similar short stories of the day or, intentionally, the exasperated cry of someone that had recognized that a fundamental flaw in his own behavior (*"the easiest way of life is the best"*) could have led to the cataclysmic ending? In other words, did the owner of the law firm come to the startling realization that the easiest way of life did not always accord with the requirements of humanity?

What is less debated, however, is the notion that the owner of the law firm represents society, and that *Nippers* and *Turkey* represent the boundaries of human behavior which a society will tolerate. In other words, that society is prepared to accept deviations and flaws, provided that they are confined and manageable. *Bartleby*, on the other hand, represents humanity itself. The *Bartlebys* of the world cannot be managed because they intrinsically contain all of the flaws of humanity. *Bartleby* prefers not to do the relentless, dehumanizing work of a machine, for his unstated reason that he is a human and not a machine – the owner cannot understand this fundamental problem and believes that *Bartleby* abuses his kindness which, to the reader, is clearly misguided.

When *Bartleby* uses the word *prefer*, he does so in order to express his humanity – sometimes to imply that he, as a human, has choices, and sometimes to imply that the choices have been made for him by the shortcomings intrinsic to his humanity.

Bartleby is also flawed in terms of his physical attributes, which progressively deteriorate, until he is of no further use to anyone and, because he is of no further use, he becomes imprisoned. Ultimately, the owner cannot understand the imprisoned *Bartleby's* depression because he cannot comprehend *Bartleby's* humanity. The owner's decision to live by his credo of *"the easiest way of life is the best"* is to ignore *Bartleby's* humanity, and to express kindness in the manner in which he believes is *easiest* – for example, by giving silver coins to the *grub-man* to keep *Bartleby* well fed. It is only after *Bartleby's* death, however, that the owner makes the fundamental and startling connection – *"Ah Bartleby. Ah humanity."*

Those of us who have had to deal with relatives or friends that have had chronically degenerative disorders will relate to the fact that these people rapidly become the *Bartlebys* of the medical world. In open defiance of all of the wonders of *modern medical science*, they seemingly *prefer not to* improve, even though this defiant preference is inarticulately expressed by the disorder rather than by the patients themselves. Nothing so aggravates an earnest medical practitioner as a passive resistance to modern medical treatment. This is a problem which, one soon learns, the medical profession, much like the owner of the law firm, has great difficulty in accommodating, particularly when *the easiest way of life is the best*. The easiest way being to assess someone's medical state, over a period of a few minutes, diagnose symptoms, and prescribe a solution to those symptoms. The missing ingredient in all this is, of course, the humanity of those who are afflicted with the symptoms, just as the missing ingredient in the story of *Bartleby* was the owner's recognition of his humanity. The owner addressed *Bartleby*'s symptoms but not his humanity.

In general, the medical world embraces the *Turkeys* and *Nippers* – those that present with transient disorders that rapidly respond to treatment, thereby providing self-gratification for the practitioners, and engendering gratitude from the patients themselves. *Modern medical systems* are really designed for *Turkey* and *Nippers* types of problems, so when such systems encounter the *Bartlebys* who *prefer not to* improve, for a sufficiently long period, and who won't go away of their own accord, they tend to become the responsibility of relatives and friends, or are eventually sent to nursing care facilities (the *Tombs*).

I tell you these things, not from an engineering perspective (which would be somewhat presumptuous with respect to such medical phenomena), but with the experience of having spent a five year apprenticeship dealing with such a medical system, while assisting in the care of my mother, who suffered from a chronically degenerative disorder.

As an engineer, I assumed that *modern medicine* meant *modern medicine* and all the implied systematic procedures to deal with those that had degenerative conditions. However, during the time which my mother was ill, I observed what went on in the *modern medical system* with some incredulity.

The first thing I discovered was that modern medicine was extremely good at dealing with healthy people (those with broken arms or those requiring knee reconstructions, for example) and it was really only sick people that had any difficulty with the *modern medical system*. Often such systems didn't work very well, and sometimes not at all. In my case, it was also particularly interesting to observe the changing attitudes with which procedures were performed as my mother's particular disorder progressed.

I did not then (nor do I now) believe that any of these attitudinal issues were a function of the individuals involved but, rather, of human nature itself – they tended to arise because *the easiest way of life is the best.*

For all of the extensive scientific and medical training that practitioners had undergone, there was no hiding their frustration when someone they had treated several months earlier (in this instance my mother) had dared to present in a deteriorated state because they had, as a consequence of their disorder, *preferred not to improve.* Self evidently, scientific and medical training had told the practitioners that this was the natural course of events. As people, however, no matter how they veneered themselves with bravado and politeness, there was an unmistakable lack of acceptance, and no hiding the fact that it was frustrating and demoralizing to have to deal with such disorders. What was the point of wasting hard earned knowledge on an ungrateful someone who *preferred not to improve?*

In caring for a relative with a degenerative condition, one quickly realized how and why the *modern medical systems* divided patients into either *Bartlebys* or *Turkeys* and *Nippers.* The *Turkey* and *Nippers* diseases were interesting and profitable to diagnose; interesting and profitable to treat; their outcomes were short and spectacular, and there was a never ending source of patients. The *Bartlebys*, after an interesting and profitable diagnostic period, rapidly degenerated into mundane pharmaceutical treatments, and profitable but seemingly unresponsive and ungrateful patients, for whom one had to assume a veneer of politeness and sympathy.

From the outset, the division of medical services, into *Bartlebys* or *Turkeys* and *Nippers*, appeared to make sense from a business perspective, if not from a health or humanitarian one.

In commencing my apprenticeship into the world of degenerative diseases, when my mother first developed her disorder, I naively believed, for example, that hospitals were places to go when one was sick. However, when one dealt with a *modern medical system*, one discovered that the last thing that hospitals wanted to deal with was sick people. It turned out that hospitals were places that wanted to have healthy people come in to undergo *procedures* and then leave. Sick people, on the other hand, were a drain on resources because they required high level nursing care.

From a business perspective, hospitals were concentrations of high-capital-cost equipment, such as medical imaging systems, operating theatres, intensive care wards, etc. In order to maximize the utilization of these high-cost facilities, a hospital was burdened with providing rooms with beds, and nursing staff to support those rooms and beds. In recent years, some clever manager with an MBA and a spreadsheet had discovered that these sundry facilities (as they had become in the *modern medical system*) were either low profit or, worse still, money losing elements of the system. Once patients stopped making use of the high-value-added services, then their occupation of a bed became a business issue because it precluded new patients from coming in and utilizing those services.

On one memorable occasion, in the early stages of my apprenticeship, I was informed, by a senior nurse, that my mother shouldn't expect to remain in hospital if all she intended to do was to lie around in bed and be sick. After all, she hadn't been making use of the facilities, and was she aware that she risked contracting a staphylococcal infection by staying there? All of which led me to ask the obvious question of why hospitals bothered with obsessive cleaning rituals if the likelihood of getting an infection was higher than in the contaminated environment of the home – which didn't have those rituals? The answer I was given by a medical specialist was very logical. The cleaning rituals were put in place to avoid spreading the sorts of infections that they threw people out of hospitals in order to avoid. During my apprenticeship, I discovered that such tautologies were an integral part of the *modern medical system*.

As if the notion of the modern hospital, composed of profit-centered medical treatment, was not enough for people with degenerative conditions to deal with, they also had to learn to contend with young interns, registrars and nurses who had suddenly realized that hospitals weren't filled with healthy and happy people. Where were all those young, good looking, healthy and happy people that got wheeled into hospital and made miraculous recoveries after being prescribed three blue pills and two yellow ones? Why wasn't the real hospital just like the ones on all the TV shows that had inspired the young medicos to take up medicine in the first place – a world where everything happened *stat*? On the TV medical shows, even the patients who didn't recover at least had the good grace to die a melodramatic and meaningful death in under 42 minutes.

In the real world, however, diseases that had looked interesting in a text book suddenly weren't all that interesting in real life – the patients who had them were often frightened, depressed, irritable, extremely rude and generally had the audacity to *prefer not to improve* despite having had two MRI scans, a PET scan and having been prescribed three blue pills and two yellow ones. Suddenly, the novice medicos discovered that the three blue pills reacted with the two yellow ones and caused major side effects that required administering four red pills, only to find that the four red ones counteracted all the benefits of the three blue ones and two yellow ones. To make things even worse, some of the ungrateful patients had the temerity to complain that the side effects of all the pills were worse than the original symptoms of the disease for which they sought treatment.

The young medicos generally believed that they had had all the right training, so they naturally subconsciously concluded that it was the patients with the degenerative conditions that were the problem and, hence, that they were trouble-makers. It was my observation on many occasions that this was the way that such patients were treated – not necessarily out of malice but seemingly out of frustration, because the young medicos had come to the realization that modern medicine wasn't all that it was cracked up to be in medical school.

The other fascinating thing that I learnt about *modern medical systems* was that, despite the fact that they were immensely complex and costly, if one was a *Bartleby*, then there were holes or gaps. As far as the medical system was concerned, these holes were only *small holes* because they were not related to *life-threatening conditions*. *Life-threatening conditions* were the euphemisms that the medical people used for cases with a high probability of litigation. When they referred to *Patient X* as having *a life-threatening condition*, they generally really meant that *Patient X* had relatives with a *litigation threatening demeanor*.

It appeared, therefore, that people with chronically degenerative disorders were *Bartlebys* because they generally did not have *life-threatening conditions* but, rather, they had *quality of life* threatening conditions. *Quality of life* threatening conditions were low on the priority list and were often just given lip-service or ignored, because the *easiest way of life is the best*. In other words, there were holes in the system. These holes were easy enough to fall into and they were often very difficult to climb out of.

By way of example, I can tell you that in one instance, my mother, who had in the latter stages of her illness become wheelchair bound, was told by one of her specialists that life would be far *easier* for her if she had a catheter fitted as part of her rehabilitation. The reasoning was that these were *trouble-free* devices which made life *easier*, and *the easiest way of life is the best*. Several days after her release from hospital, I was summoned to my parents' home, at around 7am in the morning, to be told that something had gone seriously wrong with the *trouble-free* device – obviously not *trouble* because the device was classified by the medical profession as *trouble-free*, but something. And that something was causing great distress and discomfort.

In order to remedy the problem, it occurred to me that the best course of action was to call the *In-patients* department of the hospital that had treated my mother and ask them to re-admit and assess the problem. The *In-patients* department of the hospital told me that this was only a minor matter and was actually an *Out-patients* issue, and that they would transfer me to the *Out-patients* department. The *Out-patients* department told me that the *In-patients* department must have misunderstood my request and transferred me back to the *In-patients* department, who told me that it was the *Out-patients* department who had misunderstood. Recognizing that this must have been part of a well-orchestrated medical *Abbott and Costello* routine, I decided to hang up and call the specialist.

The specialist told me that my mother's condition was only a minor matter and it was really up to either the *In-patients* or *Out-patients* department of the hospital or the district nursing service. Upon calling the district nursing service, I was advised that it was only a minor matter, and was actually a district nursing service issue, but that they were unable to do anything unless prior arrangements had been made with either the *In-patients* or *Out-patients* department of the hospital. If I had any concerns, I should address them to either the *In-patients* or *Out-patients* departments, or a general practitioner.

I called a general practitioner, only to be told that this was only a minor matter and was either an *In-patients* or *Out-patients* issue or a district nursing service issue. Or, I could also refer the matter back to the specialist. Recognizing the futility of doing another lap of the buck-passing loop, it occurred to me that the only way to quickly resolve the problem was to hire a private nursing service to come out and attend to the problem. When I called such a service and asked if a booking could be made *now*, I was told that it could. When I asked what time the nurse could come, it appeared that *now* was actually in a week. The receptionist told me that when she had booked me in for *now*, this was when the booking was made not when the nurse would come. However, I was also told that this was only a minor matter and if I wanted the problem resolved earlier, I should refer it to either the *In-patients* or *Out-patients* department of the hospital that had treated my mother, or that I could contact her specialist, or a general practitioner, or the district nursing service.

With all of the above having failed, I decided to call the emergency department of one of the local hospitals, who informed me that it was only a minor matter and if I went through an emergency room, then such an issue would be screened out by triage and it would take hours for anything to be done. I surmised, therefore, that *emergency* departments were so called because it took hours for them to actually do anything. The receptionist was, however, particularly helpful in terms of advice. Had I considered contacting the *In-patients* or *Out-patients* departments or the consulting specialist, or the general practitioner, or the district nursing service? Perhaps I could also contact a private nursing service to attend to the problem? I thanked her profusely for her advice, while verbally admonishing myself for not having considered any of these options myself.

I can still clearly remember sitting at the family dining table, surrounded by telephone books, medical business cards and pages of scribbled telephone numbers, as the clock struck up 4pm, laughing uncontrollably at the sheer absurdity of the situation. I had a PhD in engineering, I had three million telephone numbers in front of me, and I could not think of a single person or place on the entire planet that was left to call for help. Of course, what had happened was that my mother had fallen into one of those *Bartleby* holes in the *modern medical system* – her condition had been *quality of life threatening* but not *litigation threatening*. The holes had arisen because all the people in the system had been trained on the same *easiest way of life is the best* philosophy that had been applied to *Bartleby*.

By 4.30pm, it occurred to me that since no-one was prepared to accept responsibility, the next best thing to do was to just allocate it to someone and make their life hell, whether they deserved it or not. This I did by calling back the *In-patients* department of the hospital and asking for the name and position of the person on the other end of the line. I decided to make my mother's condition a *litigation threatening* condition. Rather than ask for assistance, as I had stupidly done the first time, I instead informed the poor nurse on the other end of the line that I had appointed her to manage the resolution of the problem. I also advised her that I was bringing my mother in within 15 minutes, and for her to attend to the problem, for which I held her personally responsible. I would be back to collect my mother at 5.30pm by which time, if the problem had not been fully resolved, I would return with a lawyer and she would be personally named in any litigation. As the nurse re-applied her *easiest way of life is best* approach to the problem, it was finally decided that the path of least resistance was to just fix the problem, rather than start an ongoing war. By 6pm, the issue, which everyone had informed me was only a minor matter, had been resolved, a mere 11 hours after the crisis commenced.

This was only one of many similar incidents that occurred with *Bartleby* holes. The recurring ones tended to be more related to *modern medicines* and the holes caused by the lack of coordination between specialists – the classic case of treating the symptoms rather than the humanity. One green pill would be administered by a specialist to prevent dizziness. This would cause constipation which would be remedied by two blue pills from another specialist. The two blue pills would cause nausea, which would be counteracted by three yellow pills from another specialist. The three yellow pills would cause vomiting which was counteracted by four red pills from yet another specialist. The four red pills would cause cramps which another specialist would address with five orange pills. The five orange pills would cause dizziness which, yet another specialist, would claim,

"*…had to be expected as a side effect – the bottom line is that your mother takes too many pills.*"

I guessed that this sort of high level advice was why the world had all these medical specialists. Did these people ever talk and compare pills, I wondered? Had they read Melville's book?

I cite these instances because I have heard similar cases from a number of people who have had relatives or friends with degenerative conditions, and I am sure that many others will also relate to them - they were clearly not problems peculiar to the condition with which my mother was afflicted. My mother, I discovered, had been a *Bartleby* and so had countless other people.

In my five year apprenticeship with my mother's illness, however, nothing that I had encountered intrigued me more than the medical profession's response to the most basic human condition associated with chronic, degenerative disorders. The condition was depression and the response was the antidepressant – the *doctor's little helper*. At one point, at which time my mother was bedridden, paralyzed on one side, unable to sit up even in bed, suffering from sciatic pain and a serious infection, a young medico prescribed antidepressants because my mother had clearly had developed an *attitude* problem. She had been depressed and the young medico had difficulties with this:

"And to you, this should not be so vile a place. Nothing attaches to you by being here. And see, it is not so sad a place as one might think. Look, there is the sky, and here is the grass."

It became evident that, as far as the medical profession was concerned, there was no constitutional or God-given right to depression, regardless of how dire the circumstances. The pursuit of life, liberty and happiness was sometimes constitutionally enshrined, but the right to depression was not. This sort of depression, I was informed, was clinical depression, which needed to be treated with antidepressants.

I surmised that what I had assumed was the most normal of human conditions (i.e., depression in response to a set of diabolical circumstances), was not considered medically *normal* – it was a *symptom*. Moreover, it was the defiant *symptom* of someone that had *preferred not to* be happy at that point in time, and that sort of defiance had to be snuffed out. It had to be treated with a pharmaceutical product that would engender, what I perceived to be, a highly *abnormal* response to the current human condition. Apparently, in *modern medical systems*, people who are bedridden, half-paralyzed, suffering from sciatic pain and a serious infection are supposed to be deliriously happy, I learnt – *Look, there is the sky and here is the grass.* How did I miss that?

Did the young medico seriously believe that my mother would be depressed were she not bedridden, half-paralyzed, suffering from sciatic pain and an infection? I asked.

"That is not the issue," I was told. "This is where we are now, and we have to provide the best possible treatment given the current symptom, which is depression."

I later came to realize that the antidepressants administered to patients worked very quickly and effectively in cheering up the young medicos who prescribed them, and who didn't like dealing with depressing, degenerative medical cases and grumpy patients. The doctors clearly preferred dealing with happy sick people rather than unhappy sick people. *Ah Bartleby. Ah humanity.*

Melville's book on *Bartleby* the Scrivener certainly demonstrated an enormous insight into the human psyche and its shortcomings, particularly with respect to the tolerance levels that we humans have to the human condition. The human condition is always difficult to address and difficult to manage and, so, we humans, like the owner of the law firm, choose to address the symptoms of humanity, which are far less onerous. Little wonder then that people who have chronic, degenerative conditions develop an extraordinary sense of aloneness even in a crowd. It is, ironically, the same sense of aloneness that one observes *Bartleby* enduring even though he does have friends, such as the owner of the legal firm. What is particularly interesting, however, is how broadly one can apply the lessons learnt from Melville's book in looking at what is tolerable in society and what isn't.

But how does all this discussion relate to the research in which I became involved in the area of Parkinson's Disease (PD)? Well, it does to the extent that the first thing that I learnt about PD was that it was a condition that had somehow fallen outside the boundaries of what *modern medical systems* and society preferred to tolerate – the disease itself appeared to be one of life's *Bartlebys*.

To begin with, I probably need to give you my lay-person's description of PD so that you have some understanding of its scope and impact. If you are reading this as a someone who knows nothing about the subject, then you can pretend to be impressed with my medical prowess. If you are reading this as a neurologist then you can pretend that any mistakes in my understanding aren't important and be grateful that I am not treating your patients. If you are reading this as one of the scientists, upon whose wisdom my second-hand explanation of the original facts have probably been based, then you can pretend not to sue me.

PD comes about when a particular group of cells in a localized region of the brain die off, for reasons which, at the time of writing this, are still largely unknown. There is some speculation that this cell death occurs due to a virus or exposure to toxin (we subsequently learnt in our own research that everything that medical scientists didn't understand was considered to be caused by a virus or toxin, but more about that later...). The purpose of these particular brain cells is to produce a chemical which is used to facilitate the transmission of signals from the brain to various muscles in the body. The chemical that is produced is one of a group, referred to as *neurotransmitters*, and the particular *neurotransmitter* associated with PD is called Dopamine.

The lack of the Dopamine *neurotransmitter* in people with PD makes it difficult for signals to be transmitted from the brain to various muscles, so what arises is a movement disorder – the other cognitive and mental processes are generally not affected. Without medication, people severely afflicted with the disease can find it extremely difficult to move at all because signals either don't reach muscles, or are attenuated and scrambled.

There is a broad range of symptoms that people experience to widely varying levels – to a sufferer, therefore, PD can appear very idiosyncratic. The symptoms with which many people (particularly outsiders) will be familiar are the hand tremors, twitching and flailing arms, but there are numerous hidden ones which can have an even larger impact on quality of life. These include:

- Slowness of movement (Bradykinesia)
- Problems with swallowing, digestion and bowel function
- Shrinking of handwriting size (micrographia)
- Thermoregulatory problems
- Dizziness, lack of balance, and so on.

A significant social problem of the disease is that people who have it often don't have a high level of expressiveness or responsiveness in their faces, and so are often treated as being cold, uncaring or indifferent when the real problem is one of facial muscle movement associated with the disorder.

PD is relatively common, with approximately one in every 200 people developing the disorder in older societies, so many people have relatives or friends who are afflicted. The general misconception is that the disease is actually one of older people but around one fifth of people who contract the disorder do so between the ages of 30 and 40 – these are referred to as *young-onset* manifestations of the disorder. The disease itself is generally not considered, by the medical profession, as life threatening, although the increasing severity of symptoms can be so debilitating as to cause complications that ultimately lead to death – particularly when patients become bedridden and unable to swallow food. The disease is, more fundamentally, a severe *quality of life* threatening disorder.

PD is localized to one region of the brain and so is regarded as one of the neurological disorders that is potentially amenable to a cure in the foreseeable future. For some decades, however, the symptoms of the disease have been ameliorated by the application of pharmaceutical products, which stimulate Dopamine production in the brain. Artificial Dopamine cannot be simply ingested by patients to replace the naturally generated substance, as it does not effectively pass through the blood-brain barrier. Hence, the most commonly applied treatment is a substance known as Levodopa (or L-Dopa), which is a precursor to Dopamine, that stimulates Dopamine production in the brain. L-Dopa, on its own, could be converted, by the human body, into a range of chemicals other than Dopamine, which is obviously undesirable. For this reason, pharmaceutical companies combine L-Dopa with an inhibiting chemical so that the bulk of the L-Dopa is converted into Dopamine. The combination of L-Dopa and inhibiting chemical has a range of commonly applied commercial titles, one of which is *Sinemet*. There are numerous other pharmaceutical products that are used to enhance or moderate the performance of the L-Dopa.

The introduction of L-Dopa as a treatment for the disorder was regarded as a landmark in modern medicine and some researchers estimated that usage of the drug increased patient life by more than five years, over what it might be without medication. The medication, of itself, does not cure the disease but it does delay the onset of the associated problems (chronic immobility, swallowing problems, etc.) that can lead to death from other complications.

Patients who have their medication fully active refer to themselves as being *on* and those whose medication dosage has depleted refer to themselves as being *off*. People with PD who are *on* can be highly functional in terms of mobility (to the extent where the disorder is all but invisible to a lay-person) but they can be severely dysfunctional when their medication is *off* – to the extent where they are almost completely immobile. As the disease progresses, the transitions from *on* to *off* can sometimes take sufferers by surprise and leave them immobile and unable to take medication or summon assistance, so the disease can be very frightening and stressful to those who have it.

The problem with medication is that it forces the remaining Dopamine-producing cells in the brain to increase their levels of production and has, in recent years, been considered by scientists as leading to the premature death of these cells because they are basically forced to do more work than nature intended them to do. Moreover, the brain, as a complex control system in its own right, reacts against the artificially ingested product – hence, the effectiveness of medication declines with usage, and the *on* to *off* transitions can become more and more pronounced as the disease progresses.

If, at this point, you are already thinking that the disease sounds tantalizing and that you might like to be one of the lucky one in 200 who contract it, there's more to come. As if the basic problems brought about by the disease weren't serious enough, the various forms of medication all have side effects, some of which can be quite severe and have an enormous impact on quality of life. For this reason, neurologists often give patients some latitude with their medication dosage, so that they can trade off their level of functionality against their level of side effects.

The net result of long-term usage of L-Dopa is that the brain's adverse reaction to it makes the task of controlling muscle movements even more difficult – Parkinson's patients can therefore develop a syndrome known as Dopa-Induced Dyskenesia (DID) which is a cocktail of other (even more debilitating) symptoms including muscle spasms/clenching, tics, and so on. The L-Dopa medication is also associated with psychosis and hallucinations which subsequently need to be treated with anti-psychotic drugs which, in turn, have even more side-effects.

In addition to medication, people with PD have, in recent decades, been treated with some relatively risky *let's poke around and see what happens* surgical techniques – these have the rather ominous sounding names of *thalamotomy* and *pallidotomy*. There are also surgically implanted electronic devices referred to as *deep brain stimulators* which, like the other surgical techniques, are intended to reduce the level of tremors and dyskinesia in severe patients. These treatments have varying degrees of success and, currently, all of the treatments have (at best) a transient effect which is diminished as the disease progresses.

One of the more interesting rehabilitation techniques applied to patients is the so-called *virtual reality* approach. The idea of the approach is to convert movements that normally occur subconsciously to a conscious level – for example, by asking a patient to walk from A to B on a floor which has white lines painted all over it. The feedback stimulus that this provides the brain has a positive effect on the efficiency of movement. Of course, it is somewhat impractical to expect that the entire planet will be painted over in white lines, so modern research focuses upon making virtual reality glasses that provide a similar visual stimulus. This, and numerous other rehabilitation techniques, have all been applied to varying degrees of success – generally they work better with patients who have a mild manifestation of the disease.

Young-onset Parkinson's patients are much more severely affected, in a social context, by the disease than those who contract it at a mature age. Within ten years of diagnosis, the disease becomes so disruptive to day-to-day life that a large proportion of young-onset patients are unable to continue work. As the young-onset incidence of the disease is often diagnosed between the ages of 30 and 40, this means that many people find it difficult to support their families, pay their mortgages and children's school fees, and so on. To make matters worse, because it is difficult for people with the affliction to clean up after themselves, spouses often become frustrated about the *messiness* of partners who have the disease. The sheer difficulty of doing even simple tasks, like shaving and hair-brushing, means that those without carers often look unkempt – again the issue goes back to the disorder, rather than the person, but it is clearly a more pronounced problem for younger sufferers.

Those who develop the disease at a mature age tend to be more financially secure and less dependent upon work as a means of income so have less stress in this regard. However, with an increasing propensity to go into hospitals and nursing homes (the *modern medical system*), they often do not receive the sort of care that is required to prevent rapid deterioration in their condition during hospitalization. I've already told you about my experiences with hospitals and their general aversion to dealing with sick people.

Given what I have told you about *Bartleby* and what I have told you about PD, perhaps you are now starting to see the connection. So, now that you know a little bit about the disease, you also deserve to know why it is something of a societal *Bartleby*. With any disease there are a number of issues that are of importance to those who have it:

- *What is being done to cure it outright?*

- *What medical treatment do I get today?*

- *How will my life change as a result of having the disease?*

- *How will people treat me as a result of having the disease?*

- *How much support can I count upon from society?*

On all five counts, I discovered that PD was very much a *Bartleby*.

First of all, I looked at the obvious issue of the *Holy Grail* - the outright cure for the disease. The key question was who would fund research to achieve such an objective? Apart from governments, in medical research, a key source of funding is derived from the pharmaceutical industry. However, in this instance, according to the Mayo Clinic's website, the pharmaceutical industry was getting around six billion dollars a year in the US alone from drug-based treatments for PD – not a bad business if you can get it. Multiply that figure by three to get the worldwide figure and we have an 18 billion dollar a year industry. If we assume that the average period of time that PD patients use pharmaceutical products is 15 years, then we have a business worth a total of 270 billion dollars. Funding research that would terminate a 270 billion dollar business is hardly likely to be a priority for the pharmaceutical industries of the world. This would be akin to a car manufacturer closing down some of its global activities because:

"…hell, we just felt that walking was much better for you than driving one of our cars."

One would be quite naive to think that any such move would be met with anything less than corporate resistance.

Let us now look more closely at the corporate implications of the *Holy Grail*. If one removes one's humanitarian hat and dons one's pharmaceutical corporate hat, then, leaving aside divine intervention, a curative solution can have three forms:

(i)   First of all, there is the nightmare scenario for the pharmaceutical industry – *the banana and bag of peanuts* cure, wherein some non-pharmaceutical product is found to have all-embracing curative properties. Although the likelihood of such a scenario arising is infinitesimally small, there is no doubt that even the potential for such a solution to occur would be of some business concern. A core income item disappears, with nothing to replace it, and the result is globally measured in billions of dollars of lost revenue each year. The only thing that could possibly be worse, in a business sense, would be if the same *banana and bag of peanuts* solution was found to simultaneously remove hypertension, depression and diabetes, thereby eliminating four of the big-ticket, cash flow items from the pharmaceutical industry's core business.

(ii)   A little less extreme is the *silver bullet* scenario, wherein researchers discover that a surgical/therapeutic treatment or one-off dose of some panacea can permanently cure a long-term degenerative disorder. Pharmaceutical companies, like many large organizations, maintain a portfolio of products, and plan for sunrise and sunset phases in each product line. However, this business strategy relies upon ensuring that when one product is in sunset phase, there is a new equivalent product to replace it in the sunrise phase. *Silver bullet* cures ruin this strategy if they replace life-long usage products.

(iii)   The most desirable option for the pharmaceutical world is for preservation of the *status quo* because, once a money-making machine has been built, it is far easier to just keep cranking the handle than it is to design another money-making machine. With such a scenario being unlikely, the next best option is that any research leads to new products that simply become a lifelong replacement for existing life-long pharmaceuticals. This fits in with normal sunrise/sunset business planning practices, and with the *betterment-of-mankind* spin marketing that surrounds the companies themselves.

For the most part, pharmaceutical treatments for PD have undergone regular incremental improvements over almost a half century, despite the fact that the core product (L-Dopa) remains a staple treatment for around 80 percent of patients. This ongoing improvement provides a far better quality of life for the pharmaceutical companies because it means that the newer products can be licensed when the older ones expire, thereby providing an ongoing royalty stream. In some cases, the pharmaceutical improvements also provide a better quality of life for those with PD. This is true in the case of Dopamine agonists (or agents that moderate the effect of the L-Dopa). Patients who use these newer products to supplement the basic L-Dopa can find that transitions from *on* to *off* can be less severe, and that they are *on* for longer periods – which is an extremely good outcome, for which the pharmaceutical industries need to be commended.

Countering this commendation is that fact that there appears to be very little research in terms of how to minimize the use of pharmaceutical products in the treatment of PD – the bulk of the research seems to be skewed towards increasing the amount and variety of medication. Surprising in a research sense, given that there has been scientific speculation that the use of various pharmaceuticals (while providing temporary relief of symptoms) can actually accelerate the progress of the disease. Hardly surprising from a business viewpoint, however, given who funds a significant proportion of medical research. A *Bartleby* by any other name…

Let us assume for a moment that the pharmaceutical industry has become altruistic in nature and consider the issue of developing a new pharmaceutical *cure* for PD. The conversion of research into commercially available products is difficult at the best of times. The typical formula that is applied is the 1:10:100 ratio – that is, for every dollar expended on research, ten dollars needs to be expended on development and one hundred on commercialization. In pharmaceutical areas, the ratios can be significantly larger because of the enormous costs associated with testing and approval for the use of products. The costs associated with getting a new drug into the global market can be many hundreds of millions of dollars. The ante is high and, unless there is a financial basis on which to invest in commercialization, then the business incentive is lacking. Will the pharmaceutical companies be able to charge the equivalent, for a one-off dose of a cure, to what they currently charge for, say, 25 years of conventional medication? If the answer is no, then the simple *dollar arithmetic* gives one a good prognosis for what is going to be done in a business sense.

In recent years, some governmental and benefactorial research organizations have naively postulated that, by providing more (tax-payer or benefactor) support in the high risk phases of medical research, the pharmaceutical or biotechnology companies will be more likely to take up new research and convert it into cures. The sad reality, however, is that the long-term income generated by short-term cures simply doesn't stack up against the long-term income generated by cranking out the same old drugs and upgrading them every now and then. This presents a Bartleby conundrum not only for PD but for other degenerative conditions that coincidentally form the backbone of a multi-billion dollar industry.

When we commenced our small research project, we also recognized that the diagnosis issue (or more appropriately, misdiagnosis issue), associated with PD, was somewhat extraordinary. The misdiagnosis rate was alleged to be between 5% and 25%, depending upon whether one believed the neurologists or the fPET scanning centers. After some enquiries, I discovered that the misdiagnosis rates for many other medical conditions could also be similar so this was not, of itself, unusual. But, herein was the *Bartleby* of PD – the prescription of the pharmaceutical treatment was part of the diagnostic itself. In other words, whether a diagnosis was right or wrong, the diagnosis itself would lead to an increase in sales of a pharmaceutical product for several months. PD was a *Bartleby* because even the process of diagnosis meant being subjected to the medication.

So, one didn't need to be a genius to understand why PD was a pharmaceutical and business *Bartleby*. And, even with what little I had known about the disorder, prior to my getting involved in a research project in the field, I would have guessed that, as a chronically, degenerative condition, it was also the *Bartleby* pariah of the social and medical worlds as well. Just how much this was the case, however, only became evident after our own little research program had been under way for several months, and the time came to organize participants for our doctoral research student's experiments in the field.

Our little research program would call for a control group of 10-20 people who had had no history of diagnosis of PD or, indeed, any other neurological disorders. This was the easy part, as such groups of people could often be recruited from staff or students involved with a university. The more difficult part, however, was to get another group of 10-20 people with PD to volunteer their participation.

The starting point for organizing participants was self-evident. Given that the research was outside the scope of traditional medical research, and fell into the field of biomedical instrumentation, I would need, at the very least, the imprimatur of one of the Parkinson's support groups before I could even approach any participants. I also really needed to know more about what people with PD went through on a daily basis so that we could prepare ourselves to deal with them – we were not in a medical research institute and it was important that we knew as much as possible about what we might have to deal with. A Parkinson's support group could teach us these things. However, as a researcher, there was nothing more frustrating than having to do *cold selling* of ideas to people, and that was what I would have to do with the Parkinson's support group. With industrial research, I was already past the cold selling stage when talking to companies but, with this project, it was back to square one. And, I did not like the idea of starting over in an area in which my knowledge base was almost worthless.

After doing a quick search of the Internet, to determine the local support groups and their staff, I quickly wrote down the details and telephone numbers on a notepad, with the intention of calling them a few minutes later. A few minutes later, I decided that I wasn't yet ready to do this. Cold selling was going to be difficult in its own right. From a personal perspective, it also meant re-entering all the old medical systems and tautologies that I had found so frustrating during my five year apprenticeship with my mother's ailments. If anything, the situation with PD was likely to be even worse because of the diversity of age groups involved and the broad variations in symptoms.

I finally decided that *tomorrow* would be good for starting the process. *Tomorrow* turned out to be a Friday and I decided that people associated with Parkinson's patients probably didn't want to be called on a Friday, so Monday would be better. On Monday, however, I decided that Monday was the first day of the week and people probably didn't want to be called on a Monday – mid week would be better. By mid week we were already nearing Friday again and it occurred to me that the following week would be better. Eventually, my notepad page had been completely covered in other telephone numbers and reminder messages, and I had to start the Internet search again. Needless to say, when I finally called the local Parkinson's support group, my worst fears were realized,

"And what did you say your area of specialization was again, Doctor?"

"Actually, I'm an engineer." Long, long pause (acute *Easter Island Syndrome*).

"And what was your interest, again, in speaking to our Director?"

Surprisingly, however, I did finally get through and was told that I could have an appointment with the director of the state-based Parkinson's support group, on the condition that I first met with, and spoke to, the social workers who worked for the support group. This seemed to be a fair arrangement, and so I was transferred to speak to one of the social workers. I was told that they would give me an hour of their time if I came down to see them, and that they currently supported several thousand Parkinson's patients in the state, with a suspected 20,000 being the total number.

With these numbers in mind, I assumed that the support group was therefore a large organization. However, when I was given directions about how to get there, I realized that the place was not located in a large, purpose-built facility but, rather, in a small, old brick house. The brick house, in turn, was located on the outskirts of an enormous block of land that had been the estate of a large old institution, which was still functioning as some sort of medical/nursing/rehabilitation facility, despite being encroached upon by a new housing estate. My arrival there was greeted with one of the largest down pourings of rain that we had experienced for several years, and I naively hoped that this wasn't a portent of things to come.

One would naturally have assumed that with PD being as insidious as it was, in terms of its effect on those who had it, and as common as it was in society, that support groups would be well funded. Again, a *Bartleby*. In our state, leaving aside the funding of direct medical and rehabilitation costs, the primary Parkinson's support group was given approximately ten dollars per annum per sufferer. Multiple Sclerosis, which created similar social and physical problems but had a much lower incidence level in society, had funding some six hundred times greater, per person. Why this should be the case was only made clear to me when I met with the staff from the Parkinson's support group.

I was initially welcomed with some trepidation but it was then that my five year apprenticeship in *the modern medical system* paid dividends. I knew how the hospitals, nursing homes and rehabilitation facilities functioned, and had worked out many of the *Bartleby holes* in the system, for people with chronically degenerative disorders. I also told the social workers my theory about PD being God's gift to the pharmaceutical industries of the world, and that it was His way of telling the pharmaceutical companies that He really did love them. This appeared to please them no end and, so, convinced that I already had an inkling of some of the problems their clients faced, the one hour session turned into a three hour discussion.

In the entire three hour period that I was at the support group's office, barely a minute went by when either one or the other of the two social workers was not called to answer a call from a distressed patient, who had just been diagnosed with PD, and didn't know what to do. Or, more frequently, someone who had fallen into one of those *Bartleby* holes and just couldn't get out without help. It was apparent that these people weren't just doing a job, they were also highly dedicated to those that they were trying to help.

We discussed a number of topics, commencing with mature-onset patients and working our way through to the young-onset patients. What I wanted to know was not what the neurologists assumed was going on but what actually was going on. Did these people take their medication as prescribed? This was going to be important to know for our research. What were the real complications, as opposed to the ones written on the side of medication pack (under the wonderful euphemism of *contra-indicators*)?

The picture from the coal face was, not surprisingly, quite different from what one would have gotten out of reading medical journals in the field or, as I later discovered, from talking to the neurologists themselves. The starting point from the social workers' perspective was, indeed, the void between what neurologists often assumed was going on and what actually went on. A typical scenario was painted:

"People with Parkinson's will often go through hell for months, as a result of their medication or symptoms. Eventually, however, the time comes for their next appointment with a neurologist. The day before, they will lay out their best clothes. On the appointment day, they will shower and shave and will groom themselves to look better than they have for months. They are very psyched up for the appointment; they look better and they feel better - the symptoms are often lessened when they arrive. In a half hour appointment, the neurologist will ask them how they are and they will respond that

they are well. Whether this is because they actually feel good on the day or because they fear the complications of being subjected to more pathology, scans or rehabilitation if they speak up – it doesn't matter. The bottom line is that they've told their neurologist that they are good. A few minutes after they leave the consulting rooms, the reality kicks in of another three to six months of hell before the next appointment. The adrenalin's gone, the symptoms go through the roof and, within an hour, despair and depression have taken over – that's when the telephones ring in this room. We tell them to keep a diary – always keep a diary of what is going on day by day – and give that to the neurologist. Don't just tell him how you feel on the day."

The picture that was painted was alarmingly familiar. In my five year apprenticeship with my mother's condition, I realized that I had also witnessed this scenario over and over again. Months of torment followed by,

"…good, thank you doctor."

I was quite surprised that I had not made the observation myself. Axiomatically, when symptom-based patient management was combined with a chronically degenerative condition, and a *"…good, thank you doctor"* every three months, the results were gradually building towards an inevitable crisis. And, these people were telling me that the crises were relatively common.

As I reflected on my apprenticeship with my mother's condition, it occurred to me that the body language of many of her specialists had also been along the lines of the classic Noel Coward enquiry about the state of one's health – the question is always rhetorical and nobody really cares about the answer. In thinking about these encounters in retrospect, the body language behind the *"how have you been feeling?"* question seemed to translate this into:

"I can't fix your problems so what pills do you want me to give you to get you out of here in the shortest space of time and so that you'll stop depressing me?"

Perhaps, in my mother's case, she had picked up on the body language and vibes rather than the auditory soundtrack.

One of the other questions that I had, based on my experience in seeing Parkinson's patients in a nursing facility, was about dementia. Was this related to the PD or was this just coincidental, given the age group in the nursing facility?

I recounted one incident at a nursing home, where a well-dressed lady had come into my mother's room and asked if I was her son. Thinking nothing of the tremors in her hands at the time, I replied that I was. The lady then went on to tell me how everyone was very pleased with my mother's progress since she had arrived, and how she was now more willing to sit up in an ergonomic chair, and so on. As I stood listening to this detailed diagnosis, in the best tradition of an old *Jerry Lewis* movie, two orderlies arrived to escort the lady back to her own room, which apparently she had been unable to find. I had subsequently assumed that she had dementia or Alzheimer's.

The social workers here, however, explained how Parkinson's patients had difficulty in nursing homes because their rapid limb movements were perceived as a workplace threat to nursing staff. The result was that there were always ongoing suspicions of patients being heavily dosed on medication, with some of the side-effects being confusion, dizziness and disorientation. The particularly unfortunate outcome was that these elderly patients were, indeed, ultimately treated as though they had dementia or Alzheimer's. In fact, the high level usage of some of the pharmaceutical treatments was linked to dementia. But, there was more:

"One of the problems that we have is that our elderly patients blindly follow everything their neurologists tell them even if it kills them – people in their sixties and seventies don't like questioning doctors. A few days ago, we had a frantic call from an elderly lady whose husband had had Parkinson's for some years. On the morning of his consultation with a neurologist, he had been out mowing the lawn and perfectly functional. When he saw the neurologist, he was prescribed a new medication. After a couple of days he was completely incapacitated. He was admitted to the regional hospital where he was visited by the neurologist, who told his wife that there was nothing more that he could do for them, and that her husband would have to go into full time nursing accommodation. His wife was devastated and she rang us. We called one of our colleagues who works at one of the movement disorder clinics – she sees these people every day for extended periods, so she is more in touch with what really goes on than some of the neurologists. We asked her if she had ever come across a case like this. She said that she had seen it before when patients had changed from medication X to medication Y, which was, amazingly, what had happened in this instance. She told us to contact the man's wife and suggest that he revert back to his old medication to see what happens. We called the wife and it took an enormous amount of convincing to get her to put her husband back on his old medication. She was prepared to keep going with the current medication because she thought it was her

duty to follow the neurologist's advice to the letter. We asked her to contact the neurologist to see if it was ok. Anyway, she did go back to the original medication and, within a few days, her husband was back to normal – the neurologist had already given up on him!"

Of course the really disturbing thing about this anecdote was that one immediately had the sense that it was just the tip of the iceberg. It was another one of those *Bartleby* holes, where people simply didn't know where to turn for help – somehow they fell between the cracks. The neurologists didn't seem to want to know; the hospitals didn't want to know; the general practitioners didn't want to know, and so on. Without people who had access to a broad network of contacts with wide-ranging experience in the field, the person in this case would have prematurely ended his life in a nursing home, simply because the *easiest way of life is best* and his neurologist felt that he had apparently done all that it was humanly expedient for him to do.

After a number of other such issues had been covered, the director of the Parkinson's support group came into the meeting and discussions eventually turned to the size of the local support operation and the very basic nature of the buildings. The reply was unequivocal.

"You've just entered into the land of the forgotten people of the world. It's as simple as that. You've probably walked past an average of a dozen of them in the street in the last year and have either ignored them, or assumed that they had some sort of psychiatric disorder. The fact is that if there was a children's ailment that incapacitated 20,000 to 30,000 people in this state, then there would be tens or hundreds of millions of dollars pouring in from every facet of government. Unfortunately, these people are not children; the disease is not particularly attractive or marketable to either the public or politicians, and there are very few appropriate role models on which to base the marketing."

I was quite surprised that this was actually the case, and reeled off a few famous people with Parkinson's, that I thought were all well covered by the media,

"What do you mean no role models? What about *A*? What about *B*? What about *C*? What about *D*?" The reply, however, was quite clear,

"Too old and too male. Too old. Too old and too male. And, too old and too male. That's the problem – the disease is perceived by the public to be one of older men."

"Hold on, hold on there – what do you mean too old?" I queried, "*D* is actually eight months younger than I am."

"Well that may be, but the fact is that the target demographic is people who appeal to the 16-39 year old age group. What the marketing people are telling us is – the sad fact of the matter is – to make something of interest to the target audiences, what we really need is basically a 23-year-old, blond, blue-eyed, up-and-coming, female sports star to contract the disease."

And, there it was. If *D* was already too old, and *D* was eight months younger than I, then that meant that I too had somehow become demographically undesirable. I was quite affronted by this. After all, as an engineer I had been called shallow; self-serving; indifferent; morally bankrupt; pompous; emotionally immature; bombastic; overbearing; self-righteous; a control freak; an uncaring, insensitive android, and a complete and utter waste of volume and oxygen on the planet – these were all titles that an engineer wore as badges of honor. And, we wore them with more pride than a medal-covered Russian general at a May Day parade. But demographically undesirable? This was just too much. As an engineer, I had always aspired to one day being *burnt in effigy* by some disgruntled environmental movement, but who was going to waste perfectly good fuel on an effigy of someone that was demographically undesirable?

When did one become demographically undesirable? I didn't apply for the position and I didn't remember being nominated. And, if they ever decided to make a movie of my life, did this now mean that my part had to be played by a 23-year-old, blond, blue-eyed, up-and-coming, female sports star (turned actress) in order to be demographically desirable? Is this what was meant by artistic license? And would she have the maturity and sensitivity to handle the intimate and emotionally complex lines that the screenwriters would extract from my old diaries, such as, "*change cat's flea collar*" or "*garbage day has moved to Tuesday*"?

"So, what you are telling me is that if I contract anything from this point on, then I shouldn't expect too much sympathy."

"Not unless whatever it is that you plan on contracting has already been contracted by a 23-year-old, blond, blue-eyed, up-and-coming, female sports star."

What sort of diseases were contracted by 23-year-old, blond, blue-eyed, up-and-coming, female sports stars? I wondered. *Acute Lipstick-color-mismatch-itus? Eye-liner-over-runnus Syndrome*, perhaps?

I was quite taken aback. Somehow, I had entered this discussion having just swum 3.5 kilometers and having cycled 40 kilometers, with all the enthusiasm of a *Turkey or Nippers*. I had entered feeling as though I was one of the *Turkeys or Nippers* of the world and had now realized that I, too, had become one of the *Bartlebys* instead. I had crossed the line into the land of the *Bartlebys* and, short of becoming a 23-year-old, blond, blue-eyed, up-and-coming, female sports star, there seemed to be no easy way to get back into the land of the *Turkeys and Nippers*. I was demographically undesirable. If the subject ever came up, I thought to myself, I would just have to tell people that I was *demographically handicapped* or *demographically challenged* – somehow that sounded a little better.

After the shock realization of my *Bartleby* placing in the world, the discussions turned back to the subject of getting participants for our research project and I provided an overview of what we had in mind.

"We'll help you all that we can. We'll give you contacts with all the groups in the state; we'll help you get advertisements in the newsletters and on websites, and so on. Although I don't think you'll get much interest – being a diagnostic project, and all."

"Why not?"

"These people are pretty well diagnosed as having the disease, and a lot of them have mobility problems," he said. "If you were looking at some sort of treatment, you might get more response."

What about the advancement of human-kind? I thought. What about the quest for knowledge? What about the pursuit of science and truth? What about the fact that one extremely angry research student was going to throttle me with his bare hands, if I didn't deliver him some participants? This wasn't looking good.

"Would you be prepared to come and talk to the young-onset Parkinson's group that's meeting in a few weeks time? If you made an impression, you'd probably get all the participants you wanted from there, and these people are all bright, outgoing and enthusiastic, so they're more likely to want to help you out."

"Ok," I said, "I'm happy to do that."

As one who works in a research environment, I left the meeting very much impressed with the sort of dedication that this small group had to actually assisting what was clearly a significantly under-represented section of society. And, my initial thought was that attracting participants would be a walk in the park – they would have to help – they had to consider the advancement of human-kind.

On my way back to my office, however, I stopped off at a large shopping mall to buy lunch. As I was walking back to my car, I was approached by a student, doing a master's degree in marketing, at one of our other universities. He approached me and asked if he could have a few minutes of my time to complete a survey for his research.

"What are you nuts? I haven't got time to do that. Every time you people ask for a few minutes it lasts for an hour," I replied as I quickly brushed past in order to avoid listening to him come up with some drivel about the advancement of human-kind, or the quest for knowledge.

It was not until I got back to my car, and it flashed its welcoming lights at me, that the light also went on in my head and I realized what I had just done. I had spent several hours trying to get people, who had enough problems of their own, to become involved in something that would ultimately take hours and hours of their personal time, spread over weeks and multiple visits. And, I hadn't been even prepared to spend three minutes of my own time helping someone else do the same. So much for the advancement of human-kind theory. Maybe these people with PD were nicer than I was – I was in real trouble if they weren't.

The reality dawned upon me that, unless we had more to offer the young-onset Parkinson's group than an orphan project, which was only of peripheral relevance to them, we didn't have a hope of getting any participants at all. The project was ill-conceived to begin with, and now it was apparent that it was totally screwed.

No sooner had I returned to my office when my telephone rang. It was my research student asking how I had gone in terms of getting participants. He skipped the pleasantries and simply started the conversation in his best Iranian prose:

"Are you lion or are you mouse?"

"What do you mean am I lion or mouse?" I replied.

"It's Iranian expression. Are you lion? Did you get the people with Parkinson's for the project? How did it go this morning?"

"Couldn't have gone better," I replied. Which was absolutely true, given that we apparently had nothing to offer in the first place. I didn't have the heart to tell him the part about being totally screwed. I could already see the newspaper headlines:

"Demographically Undesirable Engineer Strangled by Own Research Student – 98% of our Readers Say, "Who Cares" – Exclusive Poll"

I had to go away and think about what to do next.

Ah Bartleby. Ah humanity...

3 MOTHER OF ALL CHOP-CHOPS

Necessity may have been the mother of all inventions but when I was living at home with my parents, it was my father who was the primary procurer of many inventions – whether they had any necessity or not. Generally, these invention procurements pertained to the kitchen. All that is to say except a dishwasher which, for some still unknown reason, was shunned by the procurement process, and was always accorded the status of a device that had been the spawn of Satan himself.

Research tends to indicate that male brains typically have a higher proportion of white matter to gray matter than do female brains. It is speculated by neuroscientists that this leads to men having better spatial and mathematical reasoning than women, in general. When we men retire, that region of the brain, which is related to spatial reckoning, has to be put to some useful purpose and, in many cases, this leads to men attempting to revolutionize the kitchen environment.

Kitchen processing tasks that have seemingly been performed satisfactorily for centuries become the target of the male white matter, which hones in on them like a heat-seeking missile. Sometimes, the kitchen revolution apparently leads to friction, as was once eloquently explained to me by one of our female staff, who told me that,

"It was lucky my husband died shortly after he stopped working. If he had touched one more thing in the kitchen or had given me one more piece of advice on how I could do things better, I would have had to kill him myself. Let that be a warning to you for when

you retire and try to tinker with the kitchen — we women bring you men into this world, and we can just as easily take you out…"

In my father's case, the efficiency drive in the kitchen started innocently enough with the purchase of *Mr. Chop-Chop*. *Mr. Chop-Chop* was one of those devices that always looked like a good idea on TV at three o'clock in the morning. *Mr. Chop-Chop* was also a master of disguise because every few years he reinvented himself and reappeared on late night television under a different name. *Mr. Chop-Chop* could chop, dice and slice. However, he didn't come into our home in response to a late-night TV commercial but, rather, from a department store, because my father didn't believe in buying the *junk* that they advertised on TV.

Jobs that used to take minutes to do could be performed by *Mr. Chop-Chop* in a matter of just seconds — not including the hour and a half that it took to disassemble, wash and reassemble *Mr. Chop-Chop* and his intricate parts.

After the first two or three uses, *Mr. Chop-Chop* led a relatively lonely and unloved existence in our kitchen cupboard, until one day my father went out to buy a wedding present and returned, instead, with *Mr. Cappuccino*. This was the 1980s, and *Mr. Cappuccino* predated all the fully-automated home cappuccino machines that subsequently emerged in the 1990s.

Mr. Cappuccino's instruction manual said that he could turn out *exquisite* cappuccinos in minutes. *Mr. Cappuccino*, however, obviously felt that we already had enough caffeine in our diets because the best we ever got out of him was third degree burns by being sprayed with scalding hot steam. Amazingly, every part of *Mr. Cappuccino* was able to cause severe burns to the user and, yet, somehow, none of this heat was ever transferred to the milk or to the coffee, both of which always came out stone cold. For some years, *Mr. Cappuccino* and *Mr. Chop-Chop* shared an intimate relationship in the back corner of a cupboard until one day, when I had my own home, I inherited *Mr. Cappuccino*:

"Here, you take it — you're an engineer — see if you can fix it. It must work — why else would they sell it? We're not the only ones who bought it — they didn't make it just for me you know."

Unfortunately, they didn't have a subject called *Mr. Cappuccino Repairs*

101 at the universities where I got my degrees but, as a compassionate engineer, I decided to let *Mr. Cappuccino* live at my house. To this day, he resides at the back of a cupboard, waiting to make his debut at a garage sale, where he can move on with his life, and provide third degree burns to other unsuspecting members of our consumer-oriented society.

Mr. Chop-Chop was just a *toe-in-the-water* test at kitchen automation. The real improvements came with the all-embracing, commercial-grade kitchen mixer/blender/mincer that had attachments to do *all the jobs you hate*. We soon learnt that all the jobs we hated most were the ones associated with assembling, disassembling, washing and reassembling the attachments. So, finally, we did one of the jobs we yearned for, and threw all the *professional* attachments into the back of a laundry cupboard, where they have been gracefully acquiring a patina of rust ever since.

By the time the mid-1990s had arrived, so too had home bread making, and what better gift for my brother to give the father that had attempted to purchase almost every appliance, than the automated *home bread maker*. The gift was truly manna from heaven, particularly for a person who lived in a house that was surrounded by at least a dozen hot bread bakeries.

We soon discovered that, for less than three dollars in ingredients, and in less than three hours time (not including assembly, disassembly, washing and reassembly), we could produce a loaf of bread that was almost as good as the ones that we bought (hot) from professionals in a bakery for two dollars. The manual told us that the bread maker was:

"...ideal for when unexpected guests arrive – you'll never be caught short of fresh-baked bread again!"

Strangely enough, when unexpected guests did arrive, none of them had a spare three hours to kill while waiting for the bread maker to do its thing. And, on the one occasion that we did have guests who were prepared to wait, we didn't have the special bread making ingredients, so I had to go to the supermarket and drive past three bakeries to buy them. I decided to stop in and buy some hot bread while I was there.

I could go on to tell you about the *electric polenta stirrer* that my brother brought back from Italy as a surprise gift for my parents. No Italian home should be without one – our home was without one for all but the three and a half minutes for which it was used, before its motor burnt out. It now lives in retirement in the cupboard next to *Mr. Chop-Chop*.

Oh, and of course there was the *mess-free* automatic potato chip frying machine – the only part of the entire kitchen that wasn't a complete oily mess after using it was the cardboard box in which it came. Everything else, including most of the kitchen and the user, was covered in hot oil that sprayed all over the kitchen. The *mess-free* machine was subsequently used as a temporary paint can, before moving on to bigger and better things at a city dump.

The *mess-free* potato chip machine was designed and built by a company who prided itself in *better ideas sooner*. One of their better ideas was the *easy-clean sandwich maker*, which we also owned. It was called easy-clean because there were no parts to disassemble, wash or reassemble. Of course, because the machine could not be immersed in water, this meant that it was not only easy-clean but that it was completely uncleanable – fortunately, it only got dirty whenever it was used to make sandwiches, and when the fillings poured out over the patented *non-stick* surfaces – which was pretty much every time it was used. The *easy-clean sandwich maker* lived in the garage for a while before finding another home with some unsuspecting schmuck.

We had a few other devices that also shared the *easy-clean sandwich-maker's* wonderful, world-patented *non-stick* surface. *Non-stick* surface coatings were so called because the toxic chemicals from which they were apparently produced didn't actually stick to the metal of the cooking appliances to which they were sprayed – they usually came off after the first couple of uses. On the TV commercials, they always showed people using *non-stick* utensils to fry nails – just to illustrate how tough the coating was – of course the coating didn't adhere to the nails because they were made of the same metal as the fry pan. We didn't have much use or appetite for fried nails in the family home and, so, on the occasions the *non-stick* fry pans were used to actually fry food, we would be subjected to delicacies such as non-stick eggs – the eggs didn't stick to your insides as they were digested but the *non-stick* coating probably did. It seemed as though the only materials to which the *non-stick* coatings adhered, for any length of time, were the foods that they were meant to repel.

Many people will also be intimately familiar with another evergreen kitchen favorite – the *quick-and-easy home pasta-maker*, which was received as a gift. If one started preparing on Monday, one could have three fresh home-made fettuccini noodles almost ready by Friday – that left the weekend free to disassemble, wash and reassemble the *quick-and-easy pasta-maker*.

There were lots of other useful inventions along the way but I couldn't finish without the toaster oven that was going to *make all your other ovens obsolete*. How good is that? I thought as it arrived home – I hope people are selling all their shares in the microwave, electric and gas oven industries – for their end is nigh. After a few months of use, the toaster oven moved to a shelf in the laundry, where it currently sits, obsolete, while the other ovens are still doing their thing.

My father enjoyed cooking for others, so when he had a few guests over and I saw the giant pile of dirty dishes building up in the kitchen, I made my usual suggestion that he should buy a dishwasher, only to get the standard reply:

"What would any normal person want with a dishwasher? How hard is it to wash a few dishes? I don't know how you and your brother are going to survive in this world if you throw money away on that shit. I wouldn't take it if they gave it to me for nothing."

So, indelibly scarred by the fear of a dishwasher bringing me to penury and turning my home into a den of iniquity, I never had the nerve to have one installed. A blank cupboard sits where the dishwasher should – and it has plenty of room for *Mr. Cappuccino* to live and entertain his friends with cold coffee.

Mr. Chop-Chop; Mr. Cappuccino; the *professional kitchen grade mixer* and its attachments; the *automatic home bread maker;* the *electric polenta stirrer*, the *mess-free potato chip frying machine;* the *easy-clean sandwich maker;* the *non-stick fry-pans;* the *quick-and-easy pasta-maker*, and the toaster oven that was *going to make our other ovens obsolete*, all had one thing in common, apart from the fact that they were complete garbage – they were all obviously designed by people who didn't have to live with them or use them. And, they were all marketed as products that were an answer to the prayers of any retired male who had a higher ratio of white matter to gray matter than a female.

I cite this litany of kitchen tragedies only to highlight the fact that things which look superficially as though they will work, often don't. I also cite it as a caution to anyone who buys things that were designed by people who don't actually use them for themselves. There is often a big chasm between what looks like a good idea (even to a professional designer) and what actually is good for an end user. I used to think that this rule only applied to kitchen appliances but I later learnt that it applied equally well to pharmaceutical products, rehabilitation products and medical/surgical procedures. In one form or another, *Mr. Chop-Chop*, the master of disguise, is out there – somewhere.

When my mother was afflicted with her degenerative condition, we sought out, and often bought, numerous therapeutic products and rehabilitation devices – all of which sounded and looked as though they would work. Very few of them ever did anything. I had naively assumed that all the pills and therapies associated with various diseases had been scientifically screened, and that they were never prescribed unless the probability of them working was very high. I discovered that this was often not the case – many medical therapies only worked on a small proportion of patients, but practitioners prescribed them anyway, on the assumption that some chance at improvement was better than no chance – and anyway, it wasn't the practitioner that had to bear the cost or put up with the side-effects and inconvenience.

The medical practitioners had read all the *Mr. Chop-Chop* promises on the medical websites and in the medical magazines – some of them had even cut out the coupon that would entitle them to a free notebook computer and first-class trip to Vienna with every trial of a particular pharmaceutical product. Of course, the practitioners also had the good sense to pre-warn patients about the probability of success, so that they could have guilt-free ownership of the notebook computer and first-class tickets to Vienna, while forcing the burden of responsibility back upon the people who were in no real position to judge:

"I'm sorry, you obviously made the wrong decision when you elected to have the treatment – you must have been one of the small percentage of patients for whom it wasn't effective".

And so it went. We discovered that the medical world had an entire range of their own *Mr. Chop-Chop* products that had all been *scientifically* or *clinically* tested and proven for every conceivable disorder. Better still, the medical *Mr. Chop-Chops* had all been approved for use by swarms of government-funded medical experts and regulatory bodies. Unfortunately, as we had seen with the kitchen *Mr. Chop-Chop*, the reality often fell well short of the marketing. Even more disturbing, however, was the fact that these medical products also falsely raised the expectations of those who purchased them.

I always had a burning desire to seek out and find a few hundred other people who had attempted use the same therapeutic *Mr. Chop-Chop* products that we had procured for my mother, so that I could personally compare the success rates with the ones published by the companies that made the products. Was everyone else who tried these products a member of that same *small minority* of patients on whom these didn't work as described? I was willing to bet dollars against doughnuts that many of the products and procedures did nothing at all for any of the others either.

I need to tell you all these things as a precursor to explaining the *grand design* for our Parkinson's Disease (PD) research project, and so that you don't become overly optimistic about it at an early stage. Now that you have been introduced to *Mr. Chop-Chop*, and know that he is out there, everywhere, in many guises, you need to make sure that you remove your rose-colored glasses before reading about research – any research.

First of all, you need to understand that the overwhelming majority of research projects in universities and research institutes don't, of themselves, lead to commercial outcomes. In fact, very few research projects lead to outcomes which are even useable in the long-term – even fewer are used in the short-term, and most are never used at all.

The reality is that much of the professional research that is undertaken in the world is a means of systematically crossing off avenues of investigation – it is a process of elimination, hopefully ultimately leading to the remaining useful solution to a problem. Some researchers have great difficulty with the notion that their grand designs are little more than an item in a process of elimination – often, such researchers tend to be very creative with the truth and the data that they publish. Sometimes, somehow, despite all the screening processes, the *Mr. Chop-Chops* make it through to the marketplace and either falsely raise expectations or, worse still, cause significant detriment – lest we forget the Thalidomide disasters of the 1950s/1960s.

In perusing the Internet for the sorts of therapeutic products and treatments that had already been put forward for people with PD, I was often reminded of the empty promises of the kitchen *Mr. Chop-Chop*. As an outsider to both the disease and the medical field, I was all the more disturbed that some of the therapeutic products for PD were marketed to the medical profession and to sufferers with the same level of zeal as the kitchen *Mr. Chop-Chop*. Axiomatically, given the amounts of money associated with the various treatments, and the sheer volume of people with the disorder, the companies that promoted them wouldn't have been employing such tactics unless they actually worked.

On some of the Internet medical sites, the promoters of various PD therapies or products included *before and after* videos of how effective a particular treatment was – these were always impressive. Then, of course, much like the latest kitchen appliance, there were the testimonials – something which one would have thought that any self-respecting practitioner would dismiss out of hand as being anecdotal. However, the real world is filled with vulnerable patients who unfortunately sometimes put their faith in gullible doctors. With this in mind, and given the sort of marketing that was employed for therapeutic goods, it occurred to me that it might be a good idea for patients to ask their doctors whether they had a *Mr. Chop-Chop* in their kitchen cupboard before taking seriously any advice on therapeutic products and procedures.

You can glean from all this discussion that being an engineer is only part of what makes us innately bitter, twisted and skeptical people – this, combined with an exposure to kitchen appliances, such as *Mr. Chop-Chop*, makes us highly sarcastic as well. However, armed with this knowledge, you are now entitled to know about our doctoral research program and why being a cynic is an important asset for research. To begin with, you need to understand that a doctoral research program is essentially an apprenticeship for research. It is a means by which a person develops the ability to systematically and impartially investigate a problem, and thereby contribute to a particular field of knowledge. It is also a means by which a person develops an understanding of the key researchers and the major pieces of research in a field. Equally important is the need for a doctoral researcher to critically review his/her own work and its limitations.

It was a commonly held view amongst mature academics that the more faults and limitations that a doctoral researcher recognized in his or her work, the better the arising treatise. The reality, however, is that many doctoral researchers present their theses with the sort of promotional gusto that would make *Mr. Chop-Chop* blush with embarrassment.

Originally, the emphasis of doctoral research was to make a significant, *original* contribution to a particular field of endeavor. A hundred years ago, this wasn't too difficult to do because there were relatively few doctoral researchers around the world. I often recall the words of one elderly and eminent scientist who once remarked,

"It was easy to be an expert in my day – there wasn't all that much to know – most of what we now know to be modern Physics hadn't even been discovered…"

By the beginning of the 21st Century, however, there was quite a bit to know. And, there were typically hundreds of thousands of doctoral candidates around the world at any given time, so the notion that each one was going to make a substantial *original* contribution to the world was becoming somewhat farcical. The emphasis in a modern doctorate, therefore, is (more appropriately) to

- Assess the current state of knowledge

- Establish research directions, based upon an understanding of the work of learned peers

- Systematically extend the state of knowledge.

How far the state of knowledge is extended is somewhat subjective and always open to conjecture. Another difficulty in modern doctoral research, which didn't exist a century earlier, is the fact that there is such a vast amount of knowledge and research available, in both printed and electronic forms, that just conducting a review of literature is an awesome task in its own right – even with the assistance of advanced software packages.

In evaluating the outcomes of doctoral research, the process of examination generally requires that a candidate demonstrates a developed capacity to undertake independent, impartial research and development, and has an understanding of the limitations and flaws of that research.

In attending numerous graduation ceremonies, at various universities, it is always entertaining for me to watch the expressions on audience faces when the research areas of the doctoral candidates are read out – the audience regularly breaks into muffled titters of laughter at the esoteric nature of some of the projects. In the media, on slow news days, we regularly also experience the items about the silliness of the research topics that are often funded by various governments.

The reality is that a research project, of itself, is not the key aspect of a doctoral research program – it is a mechanism by which an individual learns how to systematically undertake research. So, it doesn't really matter whether a project relates to an international study of the strings used in tea-bags, or the frequency spectra of the laughter of hyenas. The principal issue that relates to the project is whether it is a suitable mechanism through which a person can learn the skills required to become a professional researcher.

A doctoral research program generally results in a thesis, which is typically sent to two or more internationally regarded peers for independent review. In some universities, doctoral candidates also have to have a verbal defense of their work in front of a panel of peers. In traditional doctoral programs, the research program tends to be very narrow in focus but the subject material is covered in great depth. In our particular institute, the research projects tended to be more applied in nature and so the breadth of the theses that emanated from the institute tended to be somewhat greater. We also provided a much greater emphasis on a student's independence and generally avoided the traditional master-apprentice model.

The grand plan that I had for our doctoral researcher was relatively straightforward. As I have already noted, at the time he commenced his research, there was no definitive test for PD other than autopsy. However, high-cost medical imaging techniques, such as fPET were increasingly being recognized as an accurate tool for diagnostic purposes. The problem with fPET was that while it was ok for a one-off diagnosis, it wasn't very practical for day to day testing of patients. The objective of our research would be to determine whether the human brain's electrical response to sounds (i.e., the auditory brainstem response or ABR) was an indicator of the presence or severity of PD symptoms. Moreover, could it detect the influence of medication?

In a typical PD diagnosis scenario, patients would often initially consult a general practitioner with a collection of inexplicable symptoms – loss of balance; thermoregulatory problems; tremors; uncontrolled movements of fingers, and so on. If the presented symptoms were of sufficient concern, a general practitioner would either refer a patient for conventional medical imaging (CT Scan, MRI scan) or directly to a neurologist, who could also request scans and other tests.

Having excluded a range of other probable causes, a neurologist would typically conduct simple tests for patient mobility – these tests were somewhat subjective in nature but, based upon experience, a neurologist could conclude that a person *probably* had PD. In the absence of other potential causes, a patient who *probably* had PD was often prescribed Parkinson's medication for a period of time (perhaps for months) to see how they responded – those that had a marked response to the medication were generally assumed to have the disorder. In some countries, patients who didn't like the idea of having been diagnosed with the disease opted to have an fPET scan, which provided another indicator of whether or not the disease was present.

The probability of being incorrectly diagnosed with PD was quite significant – this problem was not unique to PD but its impact on suspected sufferers was substantial. Some people who didn't have PD were diagnosed with it (i.e., a false positive), and some people who did have it were diagnosed as not having it (i.e., a false negative). Often, people who had young-onset manifestations of the disease were mistakenly assumed not to have it. The symptoms of PD are not unique – many people have low-level hand tremors but don't have any disease at all. Some people in the early stages of PD don't have the hand tremors. Moreover, other debilitating diseases can be remarkably similar in manifestation to PD – for example, Multiple System Atrophy (MSA). It was difficult even for neurologists to differentiate between these two disorders. However, patients with MSA generally didn't as respond positively to Parkinson's medication so this was one of the diagnostic differentiators that was employed.

Neurologists claimed that, with modern clinical testing and increased awareness of symptoms, the diagnostic error rate was probably under 5%. The fPET scan centers claimed that the misdiagnosis figure was still as high as 25%. So, what were the implications of getting the diagnosis wrong? Superficially, one could say that diagnosis of PD was not a particularly important issue – after all, there was no cure and the documented research suggested that the longer that patients could avoid using the medication, the better.

The problems with misdiagnosis, however, were manifold. First of all, there was the stress that patients had to endure. Some people were told that they had an extremely serious and debilitating neurological disease when in fact they didn't. Some people with the disease were told that they were fine and their symptoms were just *one of those things* – they were left with the stress of wondering why their body no longer functioned normally – until the symptoms became so pronounced and unmistakable, months or years later, that all doubt was removed. Some people who didn't have the disease at all were subjected to a period of Parkinson's medication that could last for months – and all the short and long-term side-effects that this medication entailed. And the side effects could be very severe.

Once a positive PD diagnosis was made, patients generally had regular contact with a neurologist, who would typically conduct mobility tests to determine the progression of the disorder, and discuss the medication requirements. The patients, who had some latitude in their medication, had to make some sort of subjective judgment as to how severe their symptoms were or how severe the *off* period of their medication would be – if they got it wrong, they could be caught immobile in *off* mode and unable to self-medicate. This problem of severe *on* to *off* times became more pronounced with long-term usage of the commonly prescribed drug L-Dopa. Over a period of years, as the efficacy of the medication declined and the symptoms of the disease worsened, neurologists would need to discuss with patients the possibility of surgical procedures (thalamotomy and pallidotomy) or deep brain stimulation (DBS) to provide another level of short-term relief.

In our research program, we postulated that, if it was possible to observe the presence of PD, and the severity of its symptoms, in a simple test (the auditory brainstem response or ABR) then it was also possible to have a tool to monitor disease progression and a tool to better regulate medication. Unlike the medical profession, I'd never been a big fan of diagnostic tools – I could never see the point of being diagnosed with vile diseases for which there was no cure – I therefore preferred the *ignorance is bliss* approach to life. So, it seemed to me that our *grand plan*, if not the doctoral research itself, had to go a step further. The ultimate vision should be to have a small, wearable ABR device that could either just provide feedback to patients, as to their current medication efficacy, or a device that could (ultimately) automatically regulate medication.

The machines that were used to test a person's ABR were already commonplace in hospital environments; they were technically straightforward, and reasonably low in cost (in terms of clinical equipment). One didn't need to be a genius in order to use them. Basically, they were composed of an ear-piece that was inserted in one ear; two silver-chloride electrodes (pasted onto the skin directly behind the left and right ears) and one reference electrode (pasted onto the forehead). A typical testing arrangement is shown in Figure 3.1.

The ABR machine generated audible "clicking" sounds for the patient, through the ear-piece, and then collected (and digitally processed) the electrical signals that were derived from the three electrodes. Each time a click occurred, the machine measured the resulting voltage waveform, as a function of time. A person was typically subjected to several hundred clicks, and the resulting ABR waveform was the average (ensemble) of all the individual responses.

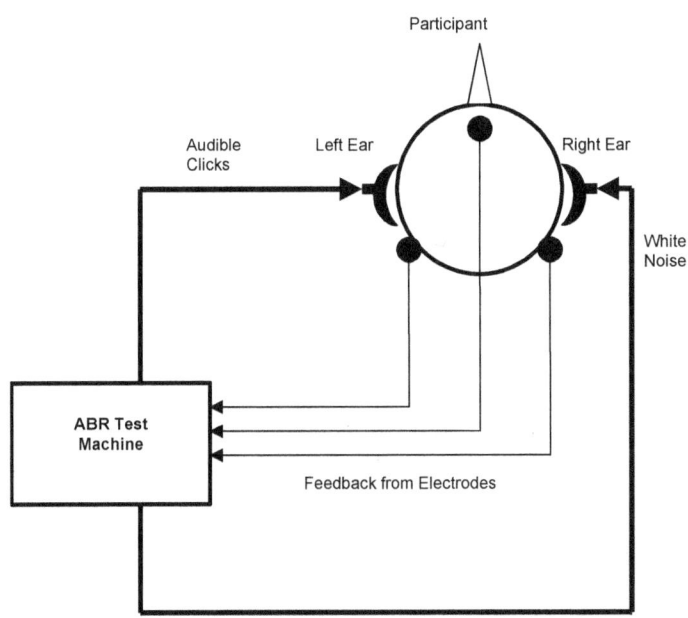

Figure 3.1 – ABR Testing Arrangement

A primary function of ABR machines in hospitals was to assess various hearing parameters in people, predominantly infants and uncooperative patients, but the machines had also been used to assess other neurological disorders – for example, people with Multiple Sclerosis presented with abnormal ABRs. A typical voltage waveform that is derived from an ABR machine is shown in Figure 3.2, as abstracted from the American Speech and Hearing Association.

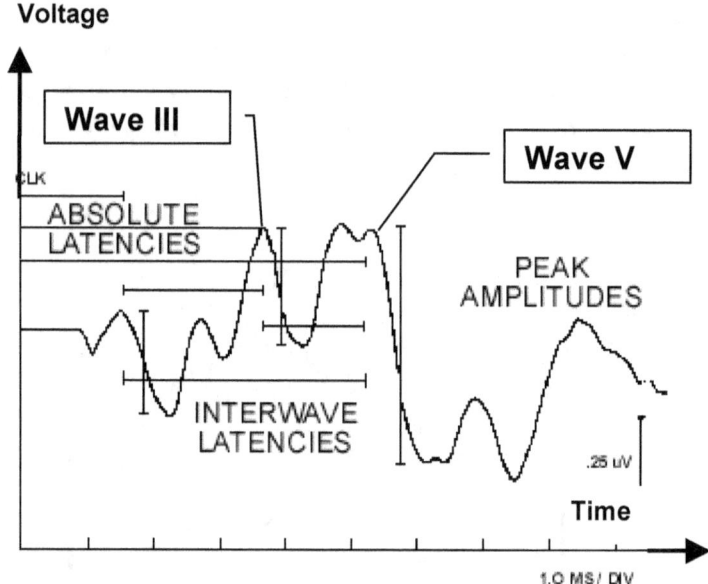

Figure 3.2 – Typical ABR Waveform

The peaks in the waveform are referred to as *waves*, and each wave is traditionally labeled with a Roman numeral – the first peak is Wave I, the second is Wave II, and so on. The timing of each wave, relative to the *click stimulus* that a person hears, is referred to as the *latency* of the ABR wave. The amplitude and the timing of each of the waves yields important information about a number of hearing parameters and, more specifically, about some of the underlying neurological phenomena that take place in the brain. Interestingly, some researchers had also discovered that various characteristics of the ABR latency could directly correlate to the core body temperature of a person. Our doctoral researcher had already been conducting work in this area before I inherited him.

There were two reasons why it was notionally possible that the ABR could have revealed information about people with PD. Firstly, there was the issue of picking up thermoregulatory abnormalities through the ABR waveform. A proportion of people with Parkinson's presented with marked thermoregulatory problems. Secondly, the amplitude of Wave V in the ABR was believed, by scientists, to arise from so-called "*post-synaptic*" activity. A synapse is a gap between two neurons (nerve cells) in the brain, and PD affects the degree to which signals are transferred across synapses because the chemical (neurotransmitter) used to facilitate this transfer is depleted. These two possible connections between PD and ABR were threadbare to say the least – but, when the research commenced, it was decided that at least it was not *impossible* that there was a connection.

The commercially-produced hospital machines that were used to measure ABR were about the size of a notebook computer, but there was no technical reason why they could not be significantly reduced in size if they were purpose-designed for personal use. The big cost factor in such machines was the value of the amplifiers that were used to scale up the signals that were derived from the electrodes – these were relatively expensive components (from a consumer market perspective, not from a professional perspective). The other issue with the commercial testing machines was that a patient had to have electrodes pasted to their skin in a rather awkward fashion and to have wires dangling all around them – a problem that could be remedied with wireless sensors if the technique proved fruitful.

Ok, so those were the basics of the idea – we subject people with PD to clicking sounds; measure their brain's electrical response (ABR) to those sounds and see how that compares to people who don't have the disorder. The other thing we needed to know was whether or not the brain's response to sounds changed as a result of Parkinson's medication or, for that matter, as a function of time of day (diurnal factors).

If it turned out that the ABR for people with PD demonstrated marked irregularities, then we would also need to know how the ABR related to the symptoms/mobility that these people had. In other words, we needed to have a measure of people's mobility (that was clinically accepted by the medical profession) and relate that to the ABR. If the mobility and ABR actually correlated, then we would potentially have a device that could provide an objective measure of a patient's condition or state of medication at any point in time. Pharmaceutical companies already modeled the effect of various drugs on the body, at a micro level, and would know how long a drug was effective in the bloodstream. In the case of PD, however, they had no objective measure of what the drug was doing to a patient in terms of his/her mobility – this was impractical to model because no two patients reacted in precisely the same way. If successful, therefore, our grand design would have been able to map patient performance against medication and time.

If we could map the performance of medication (in terms of its influence on a patient's mobility) as a function of time then, at the very least, people with PD could have better ways of self-regulating their medication. We could also extrapolate such a concept to develop a closed-loop control system that could provide automated drug infusion based upon ABR feedback.

All of the above probably sounds pretty good to you doesn't it? If you think so, then you may also be interested in purchasing a pre-owned but much-loved *Mr. Chop-Chop* that slices, dices and chops. Here is where everything gets difficult.

First of all, in order to make such a system work, we would need to start with a *gold* standard for diagnostics – in other words, how do we know that people who present to us with PD actually have it if indeed the misdiagnosis rate is significant? The answer is that the only people that we can get for such tests are those that have been *diagnosed* with the disease by a neurologist – we don't really know, until they have an autopsy, that they actually have PD. We surmised that most of our participants would be unlikely to submit to an autopsy.

Secondly, if we assumed that those who were diagnosed by their neurologists as having PD actually had it, we needed to look at the problems of the ABR itself. In order to be useful, the ABR would have to uniquely identify the presence of PD – the test wouldn't be terribly useful if it ended up showing the same irregularities for ten other disorders. This was a big problem – to begin with, ABRs were specifically designed to show up irregularities for people who had hearing disorders or Multiple

Sclerosis – would the irregularities for PD be different? What would happen if people with PD also had hearing problems? The test would be useless.

Complicating the diagnosis process even further was the fact that the disease which symptomatically appeared most similar to PD – that is, Multiple System Atrophy (MSA) – was not even well defined by the neurological community. In other words, at the time our research started, people were just beginning to define what they meant by MSA. This uncertainty made it difficult for us to test people with MSA because there was still debate about what precisely it was. Moreover, statistically, there were very few people with MSA in the community, and they didn't have organized groups, so they would be very difficult to recruit as participants for a study.

Thirdly, we had the issue of the idiosyncrasies of PD itself – would the irregularities in the ABR waveform vary with different sorts of mobility dysfunctions? Would the ABR vary significantly with different types of medication or different genders or age groups? And so on.

If, however, our ABR testing highlighted distinct anomalies for people with PD, what would need to ensue would be further research and an extensive testing program, with a wide range of subjects to determine how sensitive the approach would be. The ABR variations would need to be mapped against various medications, and so on. We simply didn't have the resources to undertake such a large scale program of tests.

Finally, in considering the development of an automated drug infusion device, there were two important issues. One was the obvious technical problem of converting a clumsy large hospital-type machine to a small, wearable device, and the other was the entire issue of legal liability as it applied to automated drug infusion devices. There were already many disorders to which automated drug infusion could be applied (diabetes being the most obvious one). The technology and devices were all available – however, for a number of reasons, the issue of product liability tended to kill off any early prospects of introducing such devices.

Over and above all these issues, was the daunting prospect of producing another *Mr. Chop-Chop*. In the cold light of day, when we started our research, we had little concept of what people with PD actually went through and whether or not they would like to have one more irritating device to deal with. There had already been numerous attempts at hare-brained devices and gimmicks to assist people with PD – rubberized sleeves to dampen flailing arm movements, and so on. The assumption with a lot of these devices was that people with a severe disorder wouldn't mind having yet another constraint and burden placed upon their lives. It was altogether possible that our *grand design*, even if it passed through all the innumerable hurdles from its vague (and thinly based) concept, could ultimately provide more nuisance value than help.

When confronted with such a plethora of issues, I decided that the obvious thing to do was to follow my own research principles and ignore all the long-term ones altogether – just focus upon the short-term issues over which we had some control. Our short-term project was to have our doctoral researcher undertake a preliminary study of the relationship between ABR and people with PD.

In order to maximize the impact of the study, we decided to have two groups – a control group, composed of, say, 15 people who had never been diagnosed with a neurological disorder, and a Parkinson's group of 15 people who had all been formally diagnosed for at least a year. In the final analysis, we would never know whether some people who were part of the control group actually (unknowingly) had PD themselves or, for that matter, whether people in the Parkinson's group actually even had the disease. These were just two basic assumptions that we couldn't avoid.

The people in the control group would just have a single ABR test performed. In the case of the Parkinson's group, we decided that maximum impact would be derived by testing them three times. On the first occasion, we would have them come in on a morning, just after they had taken their medication – we called this *AM-on*. On the second occasion, we would have them come in on an afternoon, just before they were about to take their medication. This was their medication low-point and we called this *PM-off*. On the third occasion, we had them tested an hour after they had taken their medication in the afternoon – we called this *PM-on*. On each occasion that the PD participants were tested for ABR, they would also have to undergo a mobility test, as would be carried out by a neurologist or rehabilitation specialist, so that we could assess their mobility as a function of ABR.

These tests would hopefully lead to answers to the following questions:

- When the Parkinson's group was *off*, did their ABR differ significantly from the control group? In other words, did unmedicated Parkinson's people have a different ABR to unmedicated people without the disorder?

- Did the ABR of a Parkinson's patient change with medication? If it did, then the ABR could be an indicator of the state of medication effectiveness.

- Did the ABR of a Parkinson's patient correlate to their physical mobility? If it did, then the ABR could objectively tell us the mobility of a person with Parkinson's and their medication effectiveness.

These, and other more fascinating issues that relate to far away cows and engineers, will all be revealed as you read on.

4 LIFE IN THE PAST LANE

In typical childhood development, somewhere between the ages of five and nine, children move beyond associating words with pictures and start to recognize phrases and sentences in their own right. At some stage, when I discovered reading, as opposed to connecting words with pictures, the part that impressed me the most was that every book had clearly been written just for me – it had to be, because when I read it, the voice that came out of each book was my own. By the time I was in the fifth grade, contemplating Sister Kevin's theory on those *far away cows* and their *long horns*, I was already reading 80 to 100 books a year, because all these books appeared to have been written just for me.

Somewhere in my high school years, however, I discovered that some pedagogical genius had decided that reading and enjoying books, of themselves, were undesirable traits in the educational development of humans, and that all books had to be *analyzed* and *comprehended*. Comprehension, it seemed, was reading a book and producing the exact same interpretation of it as the idiot who wrote the *comprehension* text book – even if this person had no comprehension of what the original book was about. Needless to say, as the *comprehension* content of English subjects went up, the enjoyment level associated with reading went down, and so too did the number of books read each year – usually ending with the exact same number of books having been read as was required to pass the corresponding English subject.

Even taking into consideration Sister Kevin's, all-embracing *far away cows* philosophy, it never occurred to me, at that time, that I would ultimately end up reading and writing hundreds upon hundreds of pages of text each year and writing my own books, for one reason or another.

The more that one reads and writes, the more one becomes a wordsmith, and recognizes the patterns that arise from selecting words and stringing them together. The more that one reads and writes, the more one realizes that the words and strings convey two messages – the first being the strict syntactical interpretation of the words and strings, such as can be parsed by any computer algorithm, and the second being the subliminal message that tells the reader something about the author. The more one reads and writes, the more one is able to bypass the words themselves, and unmask the subliminal messages that create an unmistakable portrait of the author. The more that one writes, the better one becomes at controlling the portrait of the author that is created.

People who are unaccustomed to writing, therefore, often end up inadvertently revealing more about themselves than they, perhaps, unwittingly realize. And, the longer the documents that people write, the more they reveal about themselves.

There were many examples of author revelation that I came across on a day to day basis as part of my work. One of these was where people, who had English as a second language, tried to impress the reader by showing their mastery of English. Of course, from the perspective of those who had English as a second language, impressing those who had English as a first language appeared to be a challenge that was based upon demonstrating how many words could be extracted from a thesaurus and forced into sentences. The sentences that were created were long and tiresome, and the words unnaturally uncommon in usage – to the extent where a reader often had to pause to decipher sentences.

Other common examples were where a person's writing style did not match up with their normal speaking style – the objective being to impress the reader. Long words were used whenever shorter ones would not only suffice but improve the reading quality of the document. These sorts of writing styles could reveal the insecurities of the author to a greater extent than the text itself ever could.

If writing is important in day to day communications, then it is critical in documenting research, particularly through theses and research papers, such as those produced at a postgraduate level. Research theses have their own particular kind of etiquette. The writer takes on the role of a humble, impartial observer and documenter of their own research. The reader is an expert who, as a devil's advocate, has the right to question, with prejudice and subjectivity, whatever has been written by the impartial author. This places an enormous burden on the thesis writer – there is little room for personal opinion or subjectivity in research writing. There is no latitude for the sort of lax speech patterns that we use in day to day life – everyday words, such as "most", "none" and "all" can no longer be used without statistical evidence to support them. "Most" requires numerical/experimental/analytical evidence of greater than 50%. "None" requires evidence of zero percent and "all" requires evidence of 100%. So, as you can see, unlike a book, every sentence in a thesis has to become an unassailable fortress because it is a defense against the subjectivities of an expert reader.

The unassailable fortress of a thesis is built up of words and strings. This takes considerable discipline in its own right because those words and strings need to unequivocally portray the author as humble and impartial, and there is no place for overconfidence or arrogance. A very important part of writing a good research thesis is in getting the subliminal message through to the reader, that the writer has become an expert as a result of what he or she has done in their research – and the difficulty is that this has to be achieved with syntax that appears humble and impartial. This is where people with poor writing skills tend to come unstuck – they display, for example, uncertainty or equivocation by choosing words and strings which, although technically and grammatically correct, do not reflect a degree of comfort with what has been presented.

If you can accept that writing one thesis will impart this level of discipline, then you can probably also accept that writing two theses will certainly hone these writing skills even further. Contributing to the writing of dozens of doctoral and master's theses will therefore impart a heightened sense of awareness of what to look for, and what to strive for, in writing:

- *Do the words and sentences chosen by the author reflect uncertainty or insecurity in what they are saying?*

- *Are the words endeavoring to cover up shortfalls in knowledge by trying to over-impress the reader?*

- *Do the chosen words reflect the sort of speech patterns that the author would use in day to day life?*

- *Do the chosen words overstate the significance of the events that have been documented?*

One eventually comes to the realization that those who have the greatest level of expertise, self-confidence and assuredness in what they do, and in their day to day lives, have a particularly interesting writing style – they tend to become masters of the understatement. Their confidence and expertise is subliminally transmitted to the reader by a balanced reporting. Personal bias is removed by juxtaposing the worst interpretations of their own opinions against the best interpretation of their opponents' opinions.

The problem with all of the precision that is associated with the writing of research theses is that, in general, as pieces of writing they tend to be somewhat sterile from a reader's perspective. Good and experienced research writers tend to have a mastery of the understatement, and bad and inexperienced research writers tend to have a mastery of the overstatement – there is little in between. So, the more that one has to read technically precise documents as part of one's work, the less interest one has in doing so for one's recreation.

In my particular case, when not reading theses, I developed an interest in reading biographies or, preferably, autobiographies – not for what they explicitly revealed about the authors through the actual text, but for what they implicitly revealed. Biographies, I discovered, tended to be very polarized, and quickly revealed whether or not the author was a sycophant or a hatchet-man for the subject of the book. For this reason, I tended to avoid them except in instances where the subject was either dead or illiterate (or both) and, therefore, unlikely to write an autobiography.

Autobiographies, on the other hand, I found to be particularly interesting from a number of perspectives. Firstly, because they were often generated by people who did not write professionally and, hence, who tended to reveal a great deal about themselves through their chosen words and phrasing. Secondly, because there was always a challenge to identify places where publishing houses had had their editors and ghost writers intervene and skew people's *personal stories* into the standard formula, which went along the following lines:

- *Childhood*

   (The *"I'm just a regular person"* section)

- *Career Ascent*

   (The *"I worked really hard and suffered to get to where I am, so I deserve it even though I feel guilty about it"* section)

- *Tragedy*

   (The *"Life sucks, and I didn't deserve this part"* section)

- *Triumph over Adversity*

   (The *"I'm really better than you ordinary, little people because I got over it"* section)

- *The Modest Hero*

   (The *"Even ordinary, little people, like you, can do what I've done"* section).

After reading numerous biographies, that had been written over some decades, it became evident that publishing houses must have conducted detailed demographic studies that had led them to conclude that this was the only formula that the public would ever accept – the odyssey of the ascent, the struggle, the triumph and the modest hero ending. This autobiographical style apparently originated from John Bunyan's autobiography and famous 17th Century book *The Pilgrim's Progress*, about which George Bernard Shaw subsequently wrote,

"This is the one true joy in life, the being used for a purpose recognized by yourself as a mighty one; the being a force of nature instead of a feverish, selfish little clod of ailments and grievances, complaining that the world will not devote itself to making you happy..."

In my reading of biographies, I surmised that whenever Shaw's famous quote (above) was invoked within a modern autobiography, it was a good indicator that the editorial staff of the associated publishing house had taken a firm hand in shaping the book and the life story into the required odyssey format.

After I had read my first dozen or so autobiographies, I learnt that there was little value in actually buying many more because they mostly employed the same formula. So, with this in mind, the second stage of my autobiographical reading phase was to just read the autobiographies in the bookstore – since there was hardly any difference between many of them, one only had to look for the minor variations in the formula anyway. This saved both money and time.

It appeared to me that during the 1980s, publishing houses had clearly worked out the business formula to publishing – that is, people don't necessarily buy books because they are good – buyers don't usually know how good a book is because they haven't read it until after they have bought it. However, during the 1980s, people had become very *brand* conscious, and so publishing houses decided that creating and/or selling brands was the key to selling books.

A brand could be a fiction author that had written a series of books, some of which had been best-sellers, or it could be a celebrity/sporting identity, for whom much of the marketing work and cost had already been borne by some other organization. By the 1990s, bookstores effectively became a front for selling brands, which were essentially book covers with a few hundred pages of content that in some peripheral way related to the brand.

In the case of *brand-name autobiographies*, much of the marketing and publicity had already been paid for by others, so the autobiography was, in effect, a license for publishing houses to print money. However, there were clearly also challenges. On the one hand, publishing houses had to satisfy their standard biographical formula. On the other hand, it was obvious that there were enormous opportunities associated with selling celebrity/sporting-identity brands, even when the content was irrelevant. In my regular pilgrimage through bookstores, I discovered that publishing houses resolved this conflict through some interesting mechanisms.

In the case of celebrities or sporting identities who had led irretrievably boring lives, or else were completely incapable of even dictating a meaningful biography to editorial staff, publishers would create coffee-table books. These could often be found in bookstores, prominently featuring the brand-name, with titles along the lines of *"My Favorite Toe-nail Clippings"* or perhaps *"The Teaspoons and Forks of My Life"*. The genius with this was that almost everyone in the chain benefited – the author from royalties; the photographers, printers, binders, publishing houses and bookstores from profits; the gift-giver from the gratitude of the recipients, and the recipients who glowed in the warmth of the thought that the gift-giver had put into the selection process. The only real losers were those who had an intelligence quotient over 50, and who attempted to read them, or to understand what the purpose of such books was in the first place.

The conventional *brand-name autobiographies* also had to somehow be forced into the standard format in order to follow the proven track record of success. For celebrities or sporting identities, the childhood and career ascent parts were straightforward. The difficulty, however, came at the point when a melodramatic tragedy had to unfold, over which the brand-name could triumph – thereby presenting the opportunity for a happy, or at least fulfilling, ending.

The problem with tragedies was that there simply weren't enough of them to go around the celebrity and sporting identity worlds, in order to satisfy the commercial publishing demand for *brand-name autobiographies*. After all, a multimillion dollar annual income often eases the pain of even the more significant tragedies. The solution, of course, was for editorial staff in publishing houses to assist in creating tragedies for the celebrities or sporting identities to overcome, along the following lines:

"...It was only after I got to the cosmetics counter and asked the assistant for a matte lipstick in Midsummer Plumb, to match my handbag and shoes, that the girl told me that Midsummer Plumb was not available in a matte. My life was in a spin. Everything that I had ever known came crashing down around me. My analyst had warned me that this would happen. I began to hyperventilate. The world started spinning around me and I collapsed to the ground, very nearly staining my designer blouse. It was my own personal Holocaust – the most devastating experience of my entire life..."

Leaving aside the trivialities of many of the lives that I discovered had been turned into books, one of the problems I encountered with reading them was that they invariably provided the reader with the editorially-compulsory, but nevertheless unconvincing and unnaturally happy, conclusion. One also finished reading them with the sense that any tragedy could be overcome provided that, like the *brand-name author*, one had tens of millions of dollars in income, prior to the advent of the tragedy, and the prospect of royalties streaming in from an autobiographical best-seller after the tragedy. This piece of information was generally excluded from the biography in order to maximize the empathy factor for the author.

Needless to say, every now and then, I found a notable exception to the standard autobiographical formula which was immensely convincing and extremely difficult to forget, even years after one had read it. A good autobiography always presented a life-changing experience for the reader. One of the most powerful autobiographies I ever encountered was Albert Facey's *"A Fortunate Life"*, which chronicled the most extraordinary life that had been led by, what the world would have considered, a most ordinary man. In Facey's autobiography, his life was very humbly presented as a *journey* – no more, no less.

Although it too was an odyssey, unlike the *brand-name autobiographies*, Albert Facey's classic, written at the age of 83 and published when he was 87 years of age, did not pander to any simplistic triumph over tragedy theme. Rather, it laid bare the journey of a very simple, uneducated man. Albert Facey had been born to immense hardship and poverty – he endured appalling cruelty and abuse after being abandoned by his mother and forced to work as an indentured servant while still a young child. During his childhood he also suffered the loss of his sister due to his mother's neglect. In his young adulthood, he was seriously wounded in one of the bloodiest battles in human history in World War I, during which time his two brothers were also killed. At the end of the war doctors had given Facey a prognosis of only a few months to live. Still he struggled on with his journey, only to suffer the loss of his farm in the Great Depression, and the loss of his son in the fall of Singapore in World War II. Albert Facey, however, battled on with his own grievous war injuries and ill health for decades before encountering his final hardship – the death of his wife of 60 years, at which point he finally distanced himself from his journey:

"I now wish to end this story. On the thirty-first of August 1977, I will be eighty-three years old – another birthday. The loss of my lovely girl, my wife, has been a terrible shock to me. I have lived a very good life, it has been very rich and full. I have been very fortunate and I am thrilled by it when I look back."

Facey laid no claim to any formula for triumph in his life, other than to have, through what he perceived to be good fortune, lived and moved on, regardless of the horrendous hardships and cruelties of fate that had befallen him in the past. One also discovered that, unlike the *brand-name autobiographies*, for Albert Facey, the process of humble acceptance and moving on did not provide the stereotypical absolution which would preclude the incidence of new hardships – right up until the very end of his life. From Facey's simple perspective, his life was fortunate because it was a life, and each new hardship that he endured was another payment that had to be made for the fortune that he had been given, and for the new adventure that it had provided him on his journey.

Facey's autobiography presented, in graphic detail, evidence that his life, like the lives of many other ordinary people, did not follow the simplistic biographical formula. There were neither Pyrrhic victories, nor enduring triumphs over tragedy, as there were in the innumerable, formularized *brand-name biographies* that had begun to sprout in bookstores like mushrooms.

Like Facey, the people that one encountered in life, who had undergone hardships, generally did not have the propensity or wherewithal to buy themselves out of them. They had to endure their hardship, and to work out how to raise children and pay mortgages and bills. Many such people were too busy enduring day to day life to write books about triumphing over tragedy. And, the irony was that many publishing houses would presumably not have a great deal of interest in publishing such books if they did, because they were not *brand-name* tragedies.

I didn't really have a problem with the formula-based, *brand-name biographies* to the extent that they provided a form of voyeuristic, soap-opera type entertainment. However, it always concerned me that they led gullible people to believe that simplistic victories would take place, if only one had *the drive* or *the commitment* or *the will to win*.

Even with this background in the limitations of commercially published *brand-name biographies*, I can tell you that my avocation in reading them generally served me very well in professional life because, leaving aside the simplistic formulae, they still provided an insight into the people who wrote them, and opportunities for opening up conversations in a broad range of areas. My philosophy was that, if one read enough autobiographies, in enough areas, then one could at least get a broad insight into what motivated people and how they perceived the world.

In the context of where we had come, in our little research project into

Parkinson's Disease (PD), this also led me to the simplistic conclusion that reading some of what people went through with this disorder would give me sufficient insight to understand their plight. I also thought that it might give me sufficient insight into the efficacy of the *grand design* for our research project to see whether there was any future in it beyond a doctoral research program. In the short-term, there was also some thought that a greater understanding would assist in recruiting participants for our project.

With only a few weeks to go before addressing the young-onset PD group, in order to attract participants for our research study, two problems had to be resolved. The first was one of research ethics approval, and the second was of what to say to these young- onset people with PD in order to encourage them to come along with us for an adventure that was not likely, of itself, to directly lead to any form of improvement in their day to day lives.

At this point, I need to note that one of the things that universities around the world have done very well, in managing research, is to introduce a range of ethical mechanisms and regulations to deal with research that involves either human or animal experimentation. At our particular university, research ethics covered all issues pertaining to research with humans – from basic questionnaires (and how data or personal information was to be stored, used and disposed of) through to actual experimentation.

We engineers have always been big supporters of research ethics, since we generally don't need to deal with them when experimenting on Toyotas or Fords – hence we encourage ethics people to make the rules as complex as possible, since we never have any intention of using them, and always have a subconscious fear of becoming victims of them. However, our come-uppance is that if we engineers ever do have to interact with humans, then we have to start from square one when it comes to ethics. What is more, ethics people (probably for very good reasons, which we engineers resent) generally don't like us engineers tampering with human beings – they have enough difficulty with the concept of engineers even speaking with other humans.

As I have already explained to you, in our research project, the basic idea was to test the auditory brainstem response (ABR) of people with PD and to compare it to the ABR of those without – and then to determine whether or not medication influenced the brain response of those with the disorder. The simplistic solution was therefore to vary medication levels and measure the brain responses accordingly. Needless to say, even the mere suggestion that engineers would have an involvement in varying prescriptive medication levels for humans would have created apoplexy in any research ethics committee. Variations in regular medication would most likely not be permitted unless participants had formal approval from their neurologists. Would any such participants go to the extraordinary length of seeing their neurologists just for the sake of participating in a study? Of course not. So – scratch one alternative.

What if, hypothetically, participants had the approval of their neurologists to vary their medication levels? Would the participants be in a state that varied from their normally medicated state while on university premises? Yes. What would happen in the event of litigation if participants, say, had an injury on the way to or from the university? Who would assume responsibility for having varied the medication levels?

What if we just asked the people with PD to come in prior to the normal time that they take their morning dose of medication – that way we wouldn't be interfering with their treatment program? What about the discomfort or rigidity that they may have getting to the university? What would happen if they travelled, unmedicated, from their homes and had an accident? Who would be responsible?

What if the researchers visited the participants in their homes? The research would not be undertaken in laboratories owned by the university. Who would be liable for any problems or costs incurred as a result of researchers conducting tests on someone else's private property? What if the tests were carried out at a hospital mobility clinic where people with PD went on a regular basis? We would require two ethics clearances – one from our university and one from the hospital involved.

Would participants' names be required for the study? No. If not, then how would participants be contacted? By a list of names, telephone numbers and email addresses. Who would retain responsibility for security of the lists and destruction of the lists at the end of experimentation? Would the data that was created, as a result of the experimentation, demonstrate any trends that could uniquely identify participants in the program? If electrical equipment was to be used in the testing process, what steps would be taken in order to ensure participant safety? Would participants be paid for their involvement? Would the researchers be trained for the experimentation program? In the event of an emergency situation arising during the course of the experiments, what processes would be in place to deal with the matter?

Would the patients be interviewed before participation? If so, what questions would be asked? Would there be any references to race? Would there be references to age or disabilities? Would the results of the interviews be documented or recorded? Would any imaging or sound recording equipment be used that could identify participants? What sort of laboratory or office accommodation would be provided during experimentation? Would participants be given paid parking on campus? Would they be provided with tea or coffee prior to, or after, experimentation?

As you can see, dealing with humans was becoming much more onerous than dealing with Toyotas and Fords. In medical research institutes, most of the above issues are relatively trivial, or non-existent, because of the presence of qualified medical experts and an infrastructure constructed around human experimentation, and recruitment for such experimentation. However, we weren't in a medical research institute – we were in an industrial research institute. So, once the medical expertise component was removed, and humans were put into the care of engineers, then the potential for litigation and disaster, arising from engineer to human interaction, was identifiable everywhere.

In our case, a colleague in the ethics committee was a qualified medical expert, with research expertise in neuroscience. He was able to provide medical advice and support in negotiating the ethical minefield that even a simple project, which connected engineers with human beings, would create. The end result was that an experimentation program would have to be developed, where participants were on the university premises; medicated as they normally would be, and that we would have to organize our timing and their timing to coincide with what we wanted to measure. It meant that we would require our people with Parkinson's to come in three times. Once in the morning, as soon as practical after their medication, and twice in the afternoon – just before their afternoon medication and again after their afternoon medication.

I need to point out here that, onerous as they are for engineers, the ethics requirements for university research are of fundamental importance to the public and protecting their interests. They are not only vital to protecting the health, safety and privacy of those who give up their time to participate in research programs, but they are also vital to protecting the emotional well-being of those to whom the research pertains. Research ethics also covers issues about how research outcomes are independently reviewed, reported and publicized – this protects those who are emotionally vulnerable from being unduly stressed by adverse findings, or by having their expectations falsely and cruelly raised by overstated research outcomes.

In the case of our research project, we felt that the compromise experimentation arrangements that were negotiated through our ethics committee were both fair and professional, keeping in mind our primary objective of protecting our participants' interests and safety. Onerous as they were, at least the ethics systems appeared to work as they should, in a university where most things didn't work at all as a result of the enveloping bureaucracy.

With the ethics issues notionally under control, it seemed that the key to getting the young-onset PD group on board was, at the very least, going to be based upon getting onto the same wavelength, and making sure that they were comfortable with the sorts of things that we were proposing. The starting point for this was clearly going to be based on reading case studies about the problems of young-onset PD people, and their lives with the disorder. This, I did, by systematically trawling through search engines on the Internet and listing organizations, chat groups, etc. Item by item, for hour after hour, I went through hundreds of personal case studies, discussion group threads, etc. and made notes.

The first observation that I had about all of the biographical information was that, unsurprisingly, given what I have told you about my views on autobiographies, it did not fit into the standard formula that was traditionally applied by publishing houses. All of these people, like Albert Facey, were clearly in varying stages of an unfinished and ongoing journey with a broad range of serious hardships and cruelties. Some of the more recently diagnosed ones were in the denial, anger or bargaining phases of their problem. Ironically, too, some of those who had been diagnosed for more than a decade were still in the anger, denial or bargaining phases.

Much of the Internet discussion related to the performance and side effects of medication, and some to the diagnostics – perhaps there was still a possibility that some diagnostic tool would reveal that there had been a mistake in the original diagnosis. Some were struggling with the idea of losing their jobs and their homes. Some were struggling with the idea of paying bills. Someone had heard that the surgical procedure called *deep brain stimulation* had remarkable results – had anyone else heard the same thing? Another had heard that they were expecting significant improvements in the technology associated with medication? Was this true? Had anyone else read about possible cures arising from the use of stem-cells? What would this lead to? Was there a cure close at hand?

The problem with absorbing the enormous amount of human dialogue that is globally generated on the Internet, particularly with respect to a subject as broad and far reaching as a disease that effects as many as one in every 200 of some populations, is that it is difficult to know where to even begin. The key issues that I summarized were categorized as follows, in no particular order:

- Diagnosis – denial and questioning

- Medication – side effects, problems and dosages

- Emotional susceptibility and rapid mood swings

- Depression

- Social isolation

- Loss of housing/accommodation

- Loss of career and employment

- Mistreatment and poor or incorrect medication in hospitals and nursing care facilities

- Destruction of family unit based upon associated social and financial problems

- Holes in the "system" – no place to go when "X" happens

- Attitudes of neurologists – disconnection between neurologists and patients

- Ambulatory and mobility problems

- Spiritual/divine guidance and/or intervention.

It was quite a depressing list of things that one might have intuitively expected, but which looked all the worse for having been assembled into a sequence that was an indictment of society and its various systems, as much as upon the disease. A lot of the problems were clearly social rather than medical. Ironically, from my perspective, the obvious item that was also notably missing from various message boards and chat rooms was a discussion of *research into* PD by those who were afflicted with it. Although the relevant Internet websites always focused upon research and newspaper extracts of current findings, the discussion groups never seemed to mirror the same level of interest. Every now and then, a passing comment would appear but I was unable to find any vigorous discussion on the subject of research, by people with PD. On the Internet sites, people with PD appeared more interested in the cure rather than the research path that led to it. Disturbingly, many were prepared to accept any touted miracle cure that might alleviate their symptoms.

I left the Internet searching one evening and considered that I would have to think over what I had summarized – I could sense the obvious patterns in what people had written but I also had a sense that I had clearly missed something that was even more obvious.

The next day, while conducting my regular *think tank* session at the swimming pool, I pondered over what I had missed. What was it about the way that young people with Parkinson's wrote that was unusual? After all the biographical reading that I had done in my life, something didn't quite fit. For some time I just couldn't put my finger on it – and then it came to me. Almost everything that they had written in their personal accounts; almost everything that I had read in discussion groups and chat rooms had the same voice to it – their lives had been written in the past tense.

That evening I went back to the various websites and chat rooms to see if this was correct. And, sure enough, it was. Whenever a person discussed their life, their reference clock appeared to stop at the last medication.

In research, writers tend to use the past tense because it gives a sense of finality and history to the work. In biographies too, because people are recounting prior events, much is written in the past tense. But, it was always my experience that people who did not write professionally, had difficulty in constantly using the past tense – this was not a normal mechanism for day to day conversation. And, yet, here in the world of young-onset PD, it seemed to be the prevailing norm. And, these people were clearly not professional writers – what was on the websites was exactly what they thought at the time, it was not an edited artwork but normal, day-to-day conversation.

Was there anything at all written in the future tense? I wondered. I trawled through as many sites as I could again. There had to be at least some sentences, such as *"Tomorrow, I am going to take my dog for a walk"* but I didn't find any on the sites that I revisited. What I did find, in many instances, proved to be even more intriguing. In situations where the future was discussed, it too tended to be discussed in the past tense, as in:

"I was thinking of completing my master's degree"

as opposed to what one would normally assume to be:

"I am thinking of completing my master's degree"

And, there was more. The other thing that I observed, in terms of writing style, was that statements would often end in question marks, such as in:

"My neurologist says that the new medication he has prescribed is working much better for me?"

I had my own amateur interpretation of why these phenomena were occurring. In the case of the past tense, it seemed reasonable that people with a chronically degenerative condition would view the past more favorably than the future. In the case of the statements ending in unnecessary question marks, there was clearly an expression of uncertainty. But, I wanted to find out what other learnt people thought.

I raised this issue with other professionals that were in the field. Since I did not come to them within anything more scientific than passing observations, I expected no more from them than just intelligent dialogue that might assist me in understanding the thought process. I casually raised the issue as part of a broader dialogue, just to see their reactions. Some of them were quite taken aback when I mentioned my observations about the writing style.

One of the psychological experts was relatively direct about the problem. His view was that, for all the modeling that was undertaken of the brain and its functions, in the final analysis, the total picture was considerably more complex than just a collection of neuronal processing devices. Changing the way that people move and function ultimately changes their place in the world and the way that people perceive their place in the world. If each day brings a new change, then it is not surprising that people's sense of identity is reflected in the way they were in the past – hence, the writing style may reflect this accordingly. Another expert's view was much the same, in the sense that she felt that personality development (that is, perceptions of self) was initiated during early childhood. Removing basic elements of coordination and movement (which contributed to a sense of self) clearly created confusion and uncertainty – for that reason people tended to reflect backwards to a point in time with which they were more comfortable.

The idiosyncratic performance of the various medications clearly provided a punctuation mark, not only in the writing style of many people with PD but, axiomatically, in their lives as well. The Internet discussions generally yielded no insights into what people with PD perceived would follow after their next medication – there were neither good nor bad predictions, nor extrapolations of lives after the next dosage.

Of course one had to take all discussions on the Internet with a grain of salt – in the final analysis, there was no way of knowing whether these reflected a random sample or, indeed, the broader views of those afflicted with PD. It could have been, for example, that these discussions were skewed towards people who had experienced extreme conditions – hence their interest in expressing themselves and their problems on the Internet. The Internet, after all, provided a large, dark room in which people could anonymously express their innermost thoughts. Nevertheless, the picture that was painted was a relatively somber one. These people, representative or not, perceived that they had very much lost their place in society and had developed a sense of aloneness in a society had not been structured to cope with this sort of disorder.

It was not altogether surprising, given their lack of interest in the future tense, that people with PD were not, at least on the Internet, vigorously discussing the future, in terms of research – other than in the sense it pertained to some form of immediate cure, which was altogether unrealistic. However, the question that occurred to me in reviewing the categorized list of discussion items that I had created was this – if a *silver bullet* cure could be prescribed today, how much of the current state of a person with Parkinson's could be undone? Although the disease was clearly a physical and mechanical one, its manifestation was far more complex. A *silver bullet* cure would never reassemble the family life that had been broken; restore the professional career that had been interrupted for years; recreate social and professional networks and ties that had been severed, or remove much of the bitterness that some of these people had developed as a result of all of these events. These people's lives had all been changed as a result of the manifestation of the disease – and, in the best case scenario, all that medical science could ever hope to do, for the people who currently had it, was to mitigate the effects of the disease itself.

Putting all these pieces of the jigsaw together didn't really assist us in our research program, and our quest for participants, but it did place into sharp relief the minuteness of any contribution that we would make to the lives of people with Parkinson's. Understanding the situation just seemed to make the task of recruiting participants even more difficult.

As all these revelations were unfolding, and I was pondering what to do next, the telephone rang and I received a call from another member of staff at the university. They had organized for a lawyer to come and see me about a potential, new research project. A week or so later, the lawyer materialized and explained that he represented a client who was a farmer. The farmer, who already had a highly sophisticated farming set up, wanted our research institute to become involved in research that would automate the cow rearing process, by monitoring the feed intake of calves and their day to day condition, including temperature, weight, and so on.

It was apparent that, just like Sister Kevin had predicted, those far away cows had finally come home to roost – or whatever it was that far away cows did. It was definitely a cow omen.

5 BEHIND THE SCENES

Sister Kevin was the first person to take us on a formal school outing to a museum. Among the many exhibits that adults, and nuns in particular, found fascinating, but were otherwise designed to bore 11-year-olds witless, was one of the structure of DNA. The exhibit was some ten feet tall and three feet wide, and it was made of wooden balls that were connected together with metal rods, in a double helix shape. The museum guide told us that this had been one of those *scientific breakthroughs* that was going to revolutionize the world, and that scientists were *on the verge* of using this DNA structure to create cures for diseases such as cancer. When Sister Kevin asked how this would occur, the museum guide told the class that DNA would be used to make pills that would one day cure such diseases. As an 11-year-old, the very thought of swallowing a pill that was ten feet tall and three feet wide, and made of wooden balls, connected together with metal rods, was an awesome concept. I guessed that they would work out the finer details of shoving the giant DNA pill down someone's throat a little later.

Sister Kevin looked somewhat skeptical and asked the guide what he meant when he said *on the verge*. The guide replied that the breakthroughs would probably come within the next few years. However, Sister Kevin continued to look skeptical about the prospects of this giant wooden structure, as anyone who had their own theorem about far away cows would be entitled to do. And, for the next three decades at least, her skepticism was well founded. When I finished high school, scientists were still *on the verge*; when I finished my bachelor's degree in engineering, scientists were still *on the verge*; when I finished my master's degree in engineering, scientists were still *on the verge*; when I finished my PhD, scientists were still *on the verge*. And, when we commenced our research project into Parkinson's Disease (PD), scientists were still *on the verge*. DNA was clearly one of those far away cows that we had already been warned about. DNA, however, taught me a great deal about science and life – not life as it was decomposed into genetic chains but life as it related to the way people behaved. DNA taught me that scientists were just as good at prevarication as anyone else. Scientists could bend the truth just as easily as they could bend light through a prism. Scientists were, in fact, masters of their own kind of magic and mystery.

Needless to say, magic and mystery have always been the most annoying of phenomena to engineers. Nothing infuriates an engineer more than not knowing how a magic trick is performed. That is to say, nothing except actually finding out how magic tricks are performed, because this takes away the enjoyment and converts the magical into the mundane. But, no matter how much we use logic and reasoning to tell ourselves that a lady hasn't really been sawn in half, there is still a minuscule, childlike part of the human psyche within us that desperately wants things to have occurred by magical means.

Engineers who keenly watch movies find the same annoying fascination with the way in which special effects are created – not knowing is infuriating – knowing makes any future viewing of the movie a completely unsatisfying experience. The eye immediately focuses upon the flaws in the computer graphics; the model building, or the polystyrene brickwork. And, we engineers know full well that the alien *Gort* didn't come from another planet to destroy the earth because he was actually the doorman from Grauman's Chinese Theatre, and because his 1950s latex suit didn't fit very well. Of course, being engineers, one of our genetically programmed obligations is to tell everyone else that we meet about such flaws and spoil their viewing of the movie as well.

As I was growing up, watching this movie magic, it never occurred to me that the painted scenery, the cardboard sets and the smoke and mirrors were all an integral part of almost every other profession as well as the movies – it was just that these other professions had different tools for creating the illusions. Only after two decades involved with research did it actually occur to me to wonder whether the magicians and movie special effects people had ever looked upon scientific researchers with the same level of naive awe with which we looked upon them – how do they do it? There must be some trick to all of this? Well, there is.

Of course the more time that one spends in a profession, the more one realizes that much of what goes on is achieved by elaborately painted facades, cardboard props and smoke and mirrors to dazzle and confuse the eye of the beholder. So, to those who have viewed scientific research in this naive awe, it is probably opportune, at this point, to take you for a tour behind the scenes and explain to you how research magic is performed. Some of the sights that you will see behind the scenes are ugly. If you are squeamish, or don't want the magic of scientific research diminished in your own eyes, then this is the time to don your rose-colored glasses or to skip to the end of the chapter.

The first thing you need to understand is that one of the big cardboard props that is employed in the research field is the notion of science, or scientific research, as a solution to our worldly problems. The smoke and mirrors are the statistics that support the research – the *good statistics* are wheeled out onto the stage whenever researchers apply for funds:

"…look how close we are to a solution…" or "…we're on the verge…"

The *bad* statistics are wheeled out whenever researchers don't have enough funds:

"…look at how far away from a solution we are because we haven't had the money…"

The entire elaborately painted research set makes for an engaging and dazzling package that is sold to either the public, business, government or a benefactorial funding body.

The harsh reality, however, is that research is a very difficult concept to sell to the public, business, government or to benefactors. In its purest sense, scientific research in a given field is largely about systematically following (and eliminating) every possible path of investigation until one reaches the correct path and a solution to a problem. Statistically, most research paths represent a dead-end and, needless to say, because there are so many paths to pursue, this process of elimination can go on for decades or even centuries with no tangible outcomes. This is of little interest to sick people who want cures within days; to a public that wants dazzling outcomes within weeks or months; to businessmen who want outcomes before the next board meeting; to politicians who want outcomes before the next election, or to benefactors who just want outcomes today, for the good of humanity as they see it.

By way of example, consider the difficulty in selling the reality of scientific research in terms of curing a particular disease. Take a good look at Figure 5.1 which shows the various stages involved. There may be a hundred starting points to pursuing that cure. Each starting point may create a pathway that has, say, ten distinct stages to it. At each stage there may be ten or more alternative options – each subsequent stage may present another ten or more options, and so on.

The end result is an exponential explosion of pathways and, in reality, there may be billions of different pathways that need to be explored between the recognition of a disease and the discovery of its cure.

Realistically, each pathway may take a year or more to pursue in a research sense.

Now, let's look at what this all means to society and for someone desperately waiting for a cure to their particular ailment. For one thing, scientists may be *lucky* and fortuitously pick the right starting point and the right sequence of paths the first time – a "one in billions" chance. This means that the time between the recognition of a disease and the discovery of its cure might be just a few years. However, if we had just one scientist looking at every possible pathway to a cure then, in the worst case scenario, the time taken to get to the cure might be billions of years – and that is assuming that we knew what the hundred starting points were in the first place.

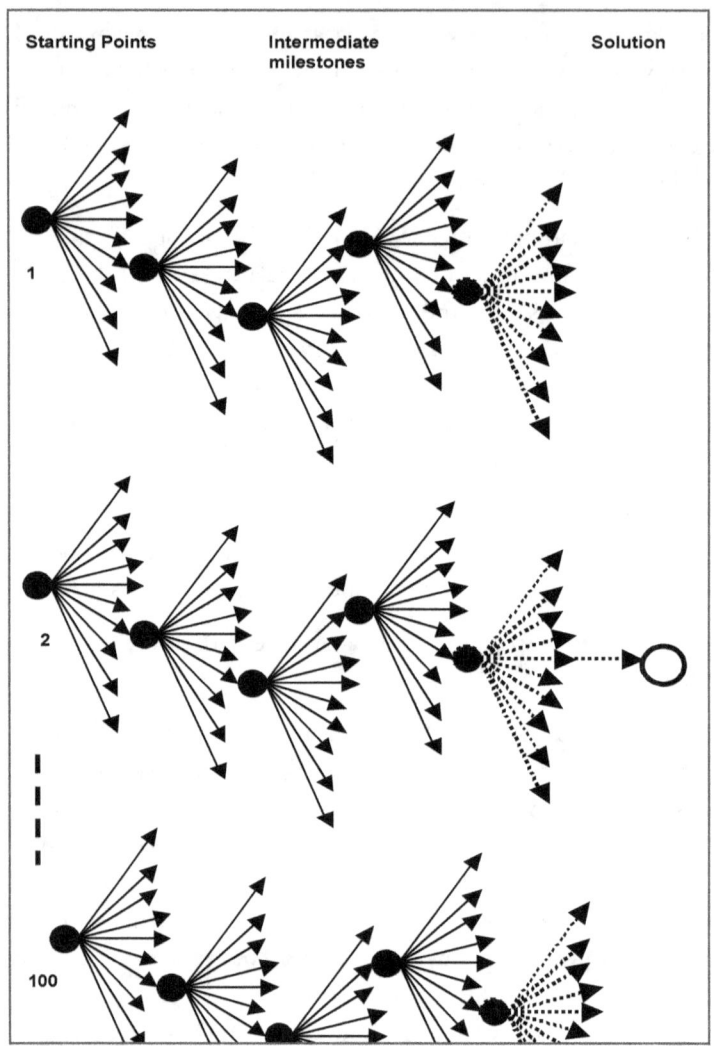

Figure 5.1 – Research Pathways

So, what is the solution to this dilemma? The solution that researchers put forward is to ask for more money and, hence, more scientists. Sounds good but then let us look at the simple arithmetic. One thousand scientists, exploring one pathway each, could still take millions of years. One hundred thousand scientists, exploring one pathway each, could take tens of thousands of years in the worst case.

How many scientists would typically be involved in research into a particular medical disorder? Typically, somewhere between a thousand and ten thousand at an international level at any given time. Just on the simple arithmetic, in a purely scientific exploration, a typical disease may take between hundreds of thousands or millions of years to fully pursue – in the worst case scenario...

Of course, scientists hope that they don't have the worst case scenario and that they don't have to go through every single possibility and path before getting to the solution. Many paths and starting points can be excluded automatically as a result of increasing knowledge as research progresses. The focus is also naturally upon excluding the number of starting points because this has the biggest impact upon the total number of paths that have to be pursued. Quite often, however, the enabling sciences and technologies that are needed for us to understand all the starting points are not even available when an exploration begins, so just excluding invalid starting points is generally difficult.

In order to find a specific example that was relevant to our discussions, and to find out what went on behind the scenes of the neurosciences research world, I trawled through book stores to locate something that would be readable for an engineer – something along the lines of *Neurology, Neuroscience and Neurosurgery for Dummies*. However, I soon discovered that these fields did not appear to be covered in the *for Dummies* series of books (an unfortunate omission, I thought) and hence I was forced to turn my search to books and research papers written by neuroscientists and neurologists instead.

Before I can explain to you the significance of what I learnt, I need to explain to you the basics of neuroscience from an engineer's perspective. To begin with, take a good look at the engineer's perspective of the human body, as shown in Figure 5.2.

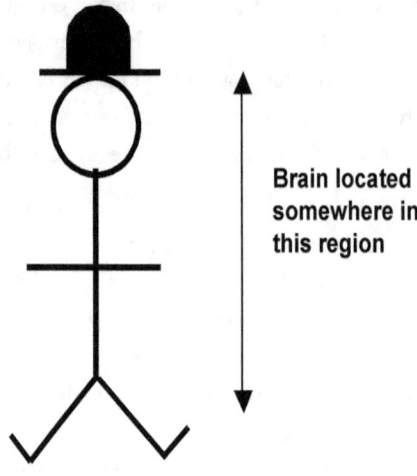

Brain located
somewhere in
this region

Figure 5.2 – Humans (as Engineers see them)

Ok, so it's probably not quite Da Vinci or *Gray's Anatomy*, but this is how we engineers view humans. You will note that I have marked out the approximate location of the brain in the diagram so that you will have a frame of reference for our future discussions. You may think this is simplistic but if you too are like many engineers, and puke at the sight of bodily organs, you will be grateful that I have adopted this engineering approach to drawing neuroscientific diagrams. Now, on to the finer details of neuroscience.

Figure 5.3 shows the human brain as engineers understand it. You will note that I have drawn the brain in a nice elliptical shape, rather than as the disgusting blob that it actually is. We engineers like to keep things neat and tidy.

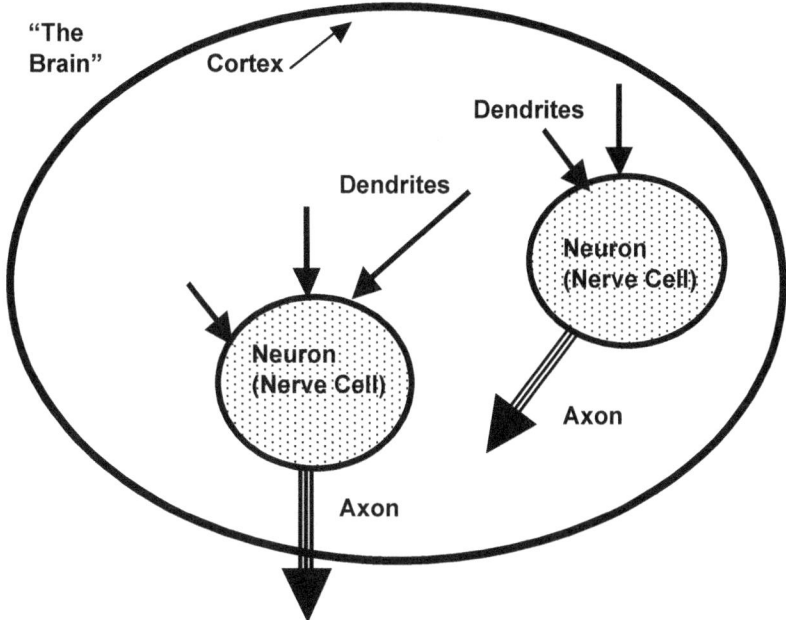

Figure 5.3 – The Brain (as Engineers understand it)

The brain actually contains billions of nerve cells (called neurons), but I have drawn just two of them for you, again in a neat elliptical shape, inside the neat elliptical brain – not to scale of course. The nerve cell body has a nucleus and cytoplasm like other cells. However, it also contains a number of inputs and outputs. The input lines are referred to as *dendrites* and the output line of a cell is referred to as an *axon*. An engineer might have labeled the input lines as *input lines* rather than *dendrites*, and the output line as *output line* rather than *axon* – but, that's the medical profession for you – never use a simple expression when a more complicated one will suffice.

Be that as it may, each nerve cell can communicate with a large number of other cells, and it can also transmit information via its axon – either within the brain or to regions outside the brain. In Figure 5.3, I have drawn one of the neurons with its axon going outside the brain because that is where our discussions are headed.

Neurological information is transmitted within the brain and around the body by what is referred to as an *action potential*, which is a voltage wave generated chemically within the cell, and which then travels along the axon. The length of an axon can vary in size from a couple of millimeters up to a meter or so in length. Information transfer along the axon is purely electrical in nature, much the same as it would be along an electrical conductor, such as copper wire.

A voltage wave travels along an axon at around 140 meters per second, which is relatively fast. The axon is covered in a myelin sheath, and this sheath is critical to the time that it takes for electrical signals to move along the axon. If the myelin sheath breaks down, then the speed at which signals travel along the axon decreases markedly – this breakdown of the myelin sheath is the basis of the disease known as Multiple Sclerosis (or MS).

Armed with all this knowledge, you are now ready to move on to advanced neuroscience as engineers understand it. Figure 5.4 shows information flowing from the brain to a muscle, via nerve cells, to initiate a movement. You will note that I have drawn the muscle in a tidy shape to complement the other tidy components. The key thing to notice about this diagram is not just the neatness of the components but, rather, the gap that exists between two adjoining nerve cells.

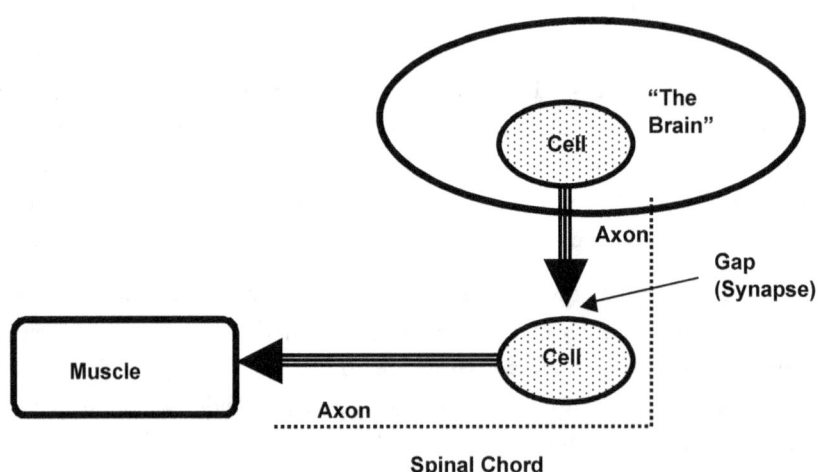

Figure 5.4 – The Brain Activating a Muscle (as Engineers see it)

Neuroscientists refer to this gap as a *synapse* because *synapse* is a much bigger word than *gap*, and if they used the word *gap* then everyone would know what they were talking about. The synapse is critical to the understanding of modern neuroscience because it is the point at which electrical conduction stops and chemical conduction begins.

In Figure 5.4, in order to transmit information across the synapse, the transmitting cell's axon fires a chemical, known as a neurotransmitter, at the receiving (post-synaptic) cell. The neurotransmitter binds to the receptors on the post-synaptic cell and this enables it to receive sodium and potassium ions, and thereby the action potential is effectively transferred, by chemical means, to the next cell. This sequence of events is important to understanding many neurological disorders and, more specifically in our case, PD.

There are a couple of other things you might need to know before we can go any further. First of all, if you have ever seen or eaten a brain, you will have observed that it has a vile, rippled outer surface (referred to as the cortex). The rippled surface of the cortex is believed to be nature's way of maximizing the surface area relative to its volume – in other words, if one took a human brain and flattened out the surface of the cortex then a couple of things would happen. To start with, the person who owned the brain would probably die, which is outside the realm of our discussions but, secondly, one would be surprised to find how large the actual area of the cortex is, given the small volume of the brain itself.

The other thing that you need to know about the brain is that the neurons near the surface of the cortex are essentially aligned orthogonal to it, and that the electrical activity that arises from groups of neurons *doing their thing* can actually be measured by placing electrodes on the scalp. This is the basis of the *electroencephalogram* or EEG. This is probably the simplest and crudest mechanism that we have for measuring the brain's activity, although the physical genesis of these signals is still not well understood. In other words, we engineers did our part by creating the measuring equipment and are still waiting for the neuroscientists to do their part.

At the other end of the technical spectrum for observing activity, there are medical imaging systems. When the neurons are *doing their thing* inside the brain, energy is consumed and a consequence of the energy requirements is that the body's metabolism varies both blood flow and deoxyhemoglobin levels – these changes are the ones that are recorded by sophisticated medical imaging systems such as functional magnetic resonance imaging (fMRI).

So, now that you have an engineer's understanding of neuroscience, you are ready to find out what I found out when I read through copious quantities of neuroscientific material, generated from tens of thousands of person-years of research, which had been conducted over two centuries.

In order to begin your tour behind the scenes, you need to know that, in the case of PD, the disorder was first formally identified by a man called James Parkinson in his essay on the shaking palsy in 1817. Why anyone would want to have a disease named after them is an interesting question in its own right. However, the point here is that James Parkinson gained notoriety for bringing together, in his essay, the case studies of people who all appeared to be afflicted with a similar disorder – you guessed it, PD.

In science, as in life, however, truth is often stranger than fiction. By the late 20th Century, researchers had come to the realization that *Case 1* of Parkinson's famous essay didn't even have the disease that subsequently came to be known as PD. It appears as though Parkinson's first case actually had the far more heinous disease, later known as Multiple System Atrophy (MSA). This disease sometimes has very similar symptoms to PD, and is still today a source of misdiagnosis. So, how is this for irony? Parkinson had a disease named after him which was so named because he had identified a collection of symptoms which turned out (at least in *Case 1*) not to have been part of the disease that was named after him!

Nevertheless, James Parkinson had actually identified, in other cases, the group of symptoms which are now related to the disorder known as PD. Needless to say, Parkinson didn't invent the disease – it had been around for thousands of years but it was his collective identification of symptoms that led to the specific naming of the disorder. James Parkinson himself identified a number of starting points for resolving the disorder and one could reasonably suggest that these were scientifically observed and pursued by himself and numerous other researchers, given the state of knowledge and technology at the time. One 19th Century path of investigation, for example, involved placing patients in vibrating chairs because it had been observed that people travelling in carriages on bumpy roads had noticed a temporary improvement in their symptoms. Needless to say, when subjected to more rigorous analysis, this path of investigation proved unfruitful. If you take another look at Figure 5.1 you will realize that the earlier that a pathway emanating from a given starting point can be excluded the better.

The initial work of Parkinson, into the disease which was subsequently named after him, provides a useful insight into why scientific research can be very drawn out – over centuries, in fact. When Parkinson commenced his investigations, the enabling technologies and sciences that were needed in order to comprehend the nature of the disease, much less cure it, did not exist, so even the meaningful starting points for scientific investigation could not be identified.

It was not until the mid 19th Century that the scientist Herman von Helmholtz performed experiments on the times taken for electrical signals to propagate, from one nerve cell to another, that the first clues pertaining to the cause of PD would eventuate – even then, the science and technology required to make the connections between Von Helmholtz's work and the disease were not available.

An assumption that many people make is that signals are transmitted from the brain, via a range of nerve cells, to various muscles, in the same way that electrical signals are transmitted around household electrical conductors, or perhaps within the data bus of a computer system – that is, by continuous electrical conduction. In other words, one might believe that the various nerve cells within the brain and throughout the body form a continuous electrical path. Of course, now that you have had the engineer's introduction to neuroscience, you know better. Von Helmholtz, however, was the one who made the interesting and pivotal discovery that the time taken for signals to propagate from one cell to another varied with temperature. This phenomenon cannot be explained by the assumption that signal transmission in the human body takes place purely by electrical means. The variation of propagation time with temperature indicated to von Helmholtz that some chemical phenomenon was also involved in the transmission of signals in the nervous system. This, albeit unrecognized by von Helmholtz at the time, was one critical starting point in the understanding of PD.

In 1875, six decades after James Parkinson's observations, a Liverpool physician, Richard Caton, first began to measure electrical impulses in the brains of living animals, and another critical element in the scientific investigation of neurological disorders began to emerge – that is, a crude electroencephalogram (or EEG) and the beginnings of the field of electrophysiology.

Another half century later, in 1920, the physiologist Otto Loewi, began experimentation with electrical stimulus of frogs' hearts, and formally determined that a specific chemical was released by nerves during the conduction process. Henry Dale and George Barger performed analogous work in England. The research revealed that von Helmholtz was indeed correct - there was no direct (conducting) electrical path between cells because gaps existed between them. The gaps were referred to as *synapses* by Charles Sherrington, and Loewi and Dale jointly received the Nobel Prize for medicine in 1936 for their discovery, which formed the basis of what is now modern neuroscience.

In 1920, however, the question that had to be answered was this – if there were gaps between nerve cells, then how could electrical signals be transferred across the gaps? It turned out that conduction of signals across a synapse could only occur when a transmitting cell released a chemical agent across that synapse. The chemical agent bound to receptors on an adjoining, receiving (post-synaptic) cell and acted like a key that enabled it to absorb conducting elements (e.g., Sodium and Potassium ions). The conducting elements therefore passed the electrical signal, by chemical means, from one cell to another. The important point to emerge here was that the transmission of signals within the human body was a combination of electrical and chemical phenomena – in other words, electrochemical conduction.

The chemicals that were released by transmitting cells, in order to enable post-synaptic cells to receive (that is, for signals to be transmitted from the brain to various parts of the body and vice-versa), subsequently came to be known as neurotransmitters. Later research also determined that there were many neurotransmitters operating within the brain, each having particular roles. Moreover, it was speculated that many neuropsychiatric diseases were caused by a too high or too low level of a particular neurotransmitter in the brain. For example, one neurotransmitter associated with the brain signals that activated muscles for human movement became known as Dopamine.

A reduction in the number of Dopamine producing cells in a particular region of the brain, known as the substantia nigra, led to a general depletion in Dopamine levels. Dopamine was an important neurotransmitter used by other regions of the brain, particularly the basal ganglia which, in turn, were responsible for control of learned movements. The lack of Dopamine led to poor signal transmission, and of course what had earlier been identified as PD. On the other hand, an excess absorption of Dopamine within post-synaptic cells was believed to be responsible for Schizophrenia. So, to some extent, PD and Schizophrenia turned out to be *duals* – one believed to be caused by insufficient Dopamine and the other by excess absorption of Dopamine.

Just why the Dopamine producing cells in the brain were injured or died off was still unknown at the time we commenced our research project, some two hundred years after Parkinson had identified the disease. The other clinical issue with PD was that the physical symptoms caused by Dopamine depletion were not unique. A number of other neurological disorders caused very similar symptoms and were a source of misdiagnosis. The disease which apparently fooled James Parkinson himself, MSA, created very similar symptoms but had an altogether different pathology. Modern differentiation between MSA and PD was based upon the use of MRI scans, which detected abnormalities in the *pons* of the brain in an MSA sufferer. However, the gold standard for PD diagnostics was still autopsy.

In my reading, I also made the interesting discovery that, in the best of old horror movie traditions, neuroscientists kept *brain banks*, which were presumably full of brains that belonged to people who had died of various neurological disorders. These had apparently been used as the basis of formal pathological testing for diseases such as Parkinson's, according to the *gold standard*. Over many decades of analyzing these brains, it appeared that as many as 10% of the people who had been diagnosed with PD actually didn't have it – they had MSA.

Of greater interest to me, as an engineer, was the fact that much of the two centuries of research into PD had been focused along a narrow range of research paths – many of these were related to the cell biology of the various nerve cells associated with the disorder. Research into the field of neurosciences determined that the many different types of neurotransmitters and neurons could be divided into two functional groups. Some were referred to as *excitatory* because they increased the likelihood of post-synaptic activity. Dopamine, for example, is an *excitatory* neurotransmitter. Others, such as gamma amino-butyric acid or GABA (I love gobbledy-gook names) could decrease the likelihood of inter-neuronal transmission of information - these were referred to as *inhibitory*. It was also determined that individual neurons could produce more than one type of neurotransmitter.

It was not until the middle of the 20th Century, however, when there was sufficient knowledge about the basic functioning of the brain, that a Dopamine depleting agent was applied to laboratory animals in Sweden, leaving them with Parkinsonian symptoms – the animals were then given a laboratory produced biological precursor to Dopamine (called Levodopa or L-Dopa) and the symptoms diminished. Of particular note was the fact that Dopamine itself could not be administered because it could not pass through the blood-brain barrier. The chemical composition of the Levodopa, on the other hand, was such that it could be infused into the bloodstream and pass through to the brain. The application of Levodopa to people suffering from Parkinson's commenced in the late 1960s and remained in use, albeit with mixed results, and no dramatic developments until the present day, despite the enormity of technological change that occurred over the same time frame.

By the beginning of the 21st Century, it was evident that the advances on Parkinson's patient outcomes, that had been achieved in almost half a century of research, were incremental rather than revolutionary. This was a common occurrence in medical science –serendipitous discovery followed by decades of incremental advances, just waiting for the next serendipitous discovery that will move the field onward.

The progression of PD treatment, although limited, occurred as a result of considerable research expenditure and effort. Many research pathways were explored in efforts to cure or better treat the disorder, and the research pathways are themselves of interest. For example, some researchers endeavored to address the idiosyncrasies of the ingested Levodopa that was used to supplement the depleted Dopamine in the brains of Parkinson's sufferers. In particular, this research had moved on to the development of drugs that diminished the actions of a particular enzyme, known as Catechol O-Methyltransferase (another really good gobbledy-gook expression, generally abbreviated to COMT). This type of enzyme prevented the ingested Levodopa from doing its job efficiently.

The benefit of the developed COMT-Inhibitors was that Dopamine drugs would last marginally longer, and that the *on* to *off* transitions for patients were potentially less severe so that quality of life could be slightly improved. This was particularly important to people as the disease progressed.

Another development involved the genetic stimulation of GABA neurotransmitter production in the brain through the introduction of a specific virus – the idea being that GABA, being an inhibitory neurotransmitter, could act to modify the frustrating tremors and rapid movements that patients suffer.

Some researchers took more of a biomedical engineering approach to the problem and developed implantable electronic devices that acted to filter out the transmission of signals that caused spurious muscle movements – this came to be known as deep brain stimulation or DBS. The problems that researchers encountered with all such approaches were the enormous idiosyncrasies of the disorder – some patients experiencing significant improvement, and many others experiencing no improvement at all.

The bulk of such developments were, in general, evolutionary rather than revolutionary, particularly in light of the half century of technological explosion that had been going on around the neurosciences. In comparison, consider how much computers had changed from the electronic-numerical-integrator-and-calculator (ENIAC) of the 1950s to the personal computer at the beginning of the 21st Century – an increase in processing speed and storage capacity in the order of trillions; size reductions in the order of millions, and cost reduction by a factor of millions. These surrounding advances in computer technology did, however, provide new avenues for neuroscientists to explore, particularly because computing gave rise to far better enabling technologies – that is, medical imaging systems and computer-based neurological monitoring and analysis systems.

A particularly interesting phenomenon I encountered during my investigation of two centuries of neuroscientific progression was that, by the 1990s, researchers had become infatuated with the emerging imaging technologies brought about by computer technology. In particular, neuroscientists had developed an enormous interest in functional magnetic resonance imaging (fMRI) and positron emission tomography (PET) scan systems in hospitals and diagnostic centers.

fMRI and PET enabled researchers to undertake what I refer to as the "pinball machine" approach to the human brain. That is, to stick a banana in someone's ear and see which part of the brain lights up, then stick a clothes peg on someone's nose and see which part of the brain lights up. The pinball machine approach to brain science could create large quantities of interesting pictures that demonstrated that one region or another of the brain was responsible for a particular function – a modern version of the phrenology theory that was popularized in the early 19th Century (and, ironically, subsequently scientifically discredited) – only this time with computer-based color images to add credence to an otherwise similar proposition. This sort of research, however, led to a greater understanding of the workings of the brain (or, at the very least, more interesting pictures of it), if not significant advancement in the treatment of neuropsychiatric disorders.

One of the technical problems with using computer based imaging techniques (such as PET) is that they generate digital images which are, in simple terms, composed of *shades of gray*. At some stage, someone or something has to determine which *shades of gray* are significant and which aren't – in other words to define thresholds by making a subjective decision and thereby convert the shades of gray into either black or white. In medical imaging this quantization generally occurs by applying a computer algorithm to the image and someone deciding that everything above a particular threshold is significant and everything below the threshold is not. The algorithm which is applied is chosen, by humans, based upon their intuitive confidence in its ability to reflect reality. Applying different computer algorithms can give different outcomes and so considerable expertise and judgment are required in interpreting the significance of the results. Putting it simply, the imaging processes do not generate 100% definitive reflections of reality, even though the quality of imaging has progressively increased with advances in technology.

The other problem with the interesting PET and fMRI images that were produced in research was that, other than adding to knowledge for the sake of having more knowledge, they didn't, of themselves, lead to any earth-shattering breakthroughs in the short-term. The images generally tended to show that the brain was a very complex structure in which control functions were both hierarchical and distributed. In other words, some parts of the brain were predominantly associated with the control of particular functions (and presumably had some form of *master* or *dominant* role) but there was also some more complex distribution of control tasks that was difficult to quantify. Moreover, some of the distributed control areas also interacted with one another. Another complicating factor was that when one region of the brain was damaged, sometimes other regions ramped up their activities to compensate. So what was the end result? In simple terms, this research led neuroscientists from the stage where they knew that they didn't know very much, to the stage where they knew more about why they didn't know very much.

In a research sense, moving from a position where one doesn't know what one doesn't know to a stage where one knows what one doesn't know is actually a significant step forward – albeit not readily useable in the short term. This is also a difficult proposition to sell to the public or research benefactors.

In attempting to put some meaning to the thousands of pages I had ingested, the question that I began to ask myself was how productive all this neuroscientific research had really been over two centuries. For one thing, I learnt that all the parts of the brain had been identified with really neat Latin and Greek names – for example, the *pons* in the brain was so called because it was the Latin word for *bridge* – this meant that the five billion non-Latin-speaking people in the world had to have the word *pons* explained to them every time the subject was raised – imagine if the *pons* had just been called the *bridge* and all that brain power wasted in the translation could have been harnessed for something more productive.

I also discovered that there had been thousands of person-years of research into the structure, organization and functionality of each of the components in the brain – culminating in the innumerable research projects involving MRI and PET scan machines, and leading to the startling conclusion that when the brain didn't work properly, it was usually because it was *broken*.

Of course, neuroscientists never actually used the word *broken* in their research papers because then even we ordinary people would understand what they were talking about. However, there were tens of thousands of pages of neuroscientific research devoted to defining *broken* and often concluding with the admission that neuroscientists didn't really understand what caused the brain to be *broken* - only that neuroscience had defined, in the most precise of Latin and Greek terms, what they thought *broken* meant.

Usually, as far as the brain was concerned, *broken* meant that either there was too much or too little of something in order for the brain to function correctly. The something was usually a neurotransmitter (e.g., Dopamine, Epinephrine, Serotonin, Acetylcholine, GABA, etc.) – sometimes the something was a tumor. When there was too much of that something, the only solution was to remove it or block its creation. When there was too little of something, the only solution was to add it. In some cases, neuroscientists weren't even sure that there was too much or too little of something – they just determined that if the level was changed then patients improved and that this was good enough. Schizophrenia was a good case in point where, in the 1950s, the drug treatment for the disease was well in advance of the understanding of what precisely happened when anti-psychotic drugs were applied.

The real problem for the neuroscientists was that removing and adding things didn't entirely fix problems from a patient's perspective. For example, anti-psychotic drugs that were used to treat Schizophrenia worked by blocking Dopamine receptors in cells. On the other hand, Levodopa added to Dopamine availability in Parkinson's patients. Both of these types of drugs led to treatments for the respective diseases and made major improvements to quality of life but neither of them actually cured the respective diseases. Both treatments had idiosyncratic effects and also created all sorts of undesirable side effects. Moreover, too much of an anti-psychotic drug in people with Schizophrenia potentially caused Parkinsonian symptoms. Too much of a Levodopa drug in people with Parkinson's potentially caused psychotic episodes.

Within these two discoveries and treatments lies one of the fundamental problems with selling the concept of research to people who fund it – for all of the science that surrounded the discoveries pertaining to PD and Schizophrenia in the 1950s, encapsulated within it was a significant component that one could only put down to luck (or serendipity, as neuroscientists prefer to call it, because it is a bigger word). The discovery that too much or too little neurotransmitter is responsible for a problem is science. The notion that simplistically adding or depleting the neurotransmitter, by pharmaceutical means, will fix the problem is largely a matter of common sense hypothesis and, above all, luck.

In the case of PD and Schizophrenia, artificially varying the level of neurotransmitter created a much better quality of life for many patients. However, in other neuropsychiatric disorders, such as Alzheimer's Disease, which is associated with the depletion of another type of neurotransmitter (Acetylcholine), the simplistic addition of an artificially produced version of the same neurotransmitter does not remedy the problem – in part, because the problem is more widespread through the brain and the reduced level of neurotransmitter is a symptom of another problem. The moral here is that, no matter how logical it may superficially appear, following two similar research paths, for two similar problems, does not necessarily yield two good solutions – one may *fortuitously* be the correct path and the other may *unfortunately* be another of many incorrect paths.

Another interesting observation which I made in relation to neuroscientific work over the centuries was that it was predominantly based on chemical, biochemical and biological expertise and analysis, rather than on expertise in the physics and mathematics that are commonly applied in engineering and technology. So, what were the consequences of this constraint that was imposed by the natural historical development of the field?

For one thing, the constraint that was imposed by the limited skill sets of those undertaking the research meant that scientists had defined the problem of understanding the brain and its disorders at a micro level. In other words, they started with molecules and cells, and tried to work their micro understanding upwards to the entire brain. This was a *bottom-up* approach to research and, if the brain had turned out to be a simple biochemical device, then the chosen research pathway might have quickly yielded solutions to many problems. However, as luck would have it, the brain turned out to be an immensely complex device and the chosen research paths could not readily be extrapolated upwards.

In retrospect (and retrospective observations are always cheap and plentiful), in terms of remedying problems, the *bottom-up* pathways that had been pursued in neuroscientific research were analogous to a mechanic endeavoring to repair a car by starting with the atomic structure of the materials used to build it – eventually the mechanic may arrive at the solution to the problem, which may be to replace a broken spark-plug, but this may take several thousand years – a luxury which we seldom accord to mechanics, especially when we pay them on an hourly basis.

Moreover, in the car repair analogy, if the mechanic acquires an intimate understanding of how each atom is connected to other atoms, will he ever be able to step back and assemble the bigger picture? Or, will he just have a massively complex picture of an atomic structure, rather than a picture of an engine that has a broken spark-plug? This may sound silly but it is critically important because it is all about the way we look at scientific problems – sooner or later there comes a time when new paradigms are needed. In reading the scientific research, it became evident that, by the beginning of the 21st Century, new paradigms were desperately needed in the neurosciences and these would not necessarily be solely based upon cell biology and biochemistry, important as both these fields were to understanding the problem.

In other areas of science, physicists were quick to recognize that looking at individual molecules would never explain the behavior of certain phenomena – for example, gases. So they developed a new paradigm – they looked at the phenomena of gases at a higher level and developed the gas laws which are in use today. Neuroscientific research had reached a similar plateau with its existing paradigm – a micro picture which could not readily be extrapolated into a workable macro picture.

Not surprisingly, some researchers recognized that the *bottom-up* approach had plateaued and turned to a *top-down* approach, based upon images of the brain acquired from fMRI and PET scans – the pinball machine approach. This was the other extreme and tended to create macro pictures that were too big in scale to facilitate detailed understanding. How much do scientists really learn when they discover that a particular region of the brain lights up when they stick a banana in someone's ear? The fMRI and PET scans could show functionality but it was a complex task to work downwards back to the micro issues. Returning to the car repair analogy, this sort of research was very much like trying to fix a car by taking a satellite photo of it from space – it may be possible to tell that the car has wheels and an engine, but which part of the engine is broken and how can one diagnose it from that distance?

After two centuries of neuroscientific research, it was a difficult task to even bring the *bottom-up* and the *top-down* pieces of research knowledge together. Even a complete outsider to the field, such as myself, could see that there was an enormous void between them. In a sense, it was akin to having the mechanic who is trying to fix a car by looking at its atomic structure consulting with the mechanic who is trying to fix the same car by taking satellite photos of it. They have no common language and both need to be retrained in order to even be able to communicate with one another. Clearly, however, the solution had to be to find people who could take a view somewhere in between the two extremes.

The neuroscientists might well tell us that the reason that cars are so readily fixed is because they are simple devices compared to the enormously complex brain. Of course, if we engineers took the same atom by atom approach to research, then we would argue that the same complexity is true of a gearbox or refrigerator or a washing machine, much less a modern microprocessor chip.

The problem, I observed, is that we engineers view the world very differently to neuroscientists. In fact, the development of the microprocessor chip, which is the closest analogy that we engineers have to the human brain, shows the different thought processes that are involved. The original science (that is, semiconductor physics), upon which the original transistor of the 1940s was based, quickly gave way to a level of abstraction that was one step up. And that level of abstraction led to the next level, and so on. Transistors formed digital logic circuits; digital logic circuits formed counters, memory and mathematical reckoning circuits, and the combination of these formed a microprocessor. The microprocessor formed a functional block for the next level of abstraction (the computer) and the computer formed a functional block for software development.

There are two significant outcomes that arose from this stepwise increase in understanding of electronics and computers. Firstly, modern computer programmers do not need to be concerned with semiconductor physics to do their jobs. Secondly, within the computer and electronics industries, it is possible to find a spectrum of people with skills ranging from semiconductor physics (*bottom-up*) to software development (*top-down*) – and most of these people can communicate with one another. This is no small thing. This enormous evolution in abstraction occurred in the space of only half a century.

In the neurosciences, which were always mired in the mysteries of medical research, there appeared to be no analogous evolution over the same period. Neuroscientists argue (perhaps correctly) that the reason that they cannot do the same thing with the brain is that one cannot simply scale up the level of abstraction in the thought process – in other words, that the brain is not merely a collection of bits and pieces that bolt together in order to function.

In terms of the neurosciences, however, bridging the void between the *bottom-up* and *top-down* researchers involves creating specialists who have expertise in biology, chemistry, biochemistry, mathematics and physics to create meaningful models of the brain. Unfortunately, the languages of mathematics/physics based researchers and biology/chemistry based researchers are completely different. Often it is the case that one discipline is not even aware that their skills can be applied to another area, or that the skills from another discipline can be applied to their own area. Moreover, there is a natural tendency in research to keep pursuing a narrow area even if that area proves somewhat unproductive at a particular point in time. However, by the beginning of the 21st Century, there was a small and emerging set of researchers that endeavored to bridge the *bottom-up* and *top-down* approaches in neuroscientific research.

In terms of the *bottom-up* biology/chemistry based researchers, and their ongoing foray in to PD, the crème-de-la-crème of research pathways that had captured their attention involved the use of stem-cells to replace the damaged cells that would normally produce Dopamine in the brain. Stem-cells were effectively *unconfigured* human cells that could be *configured* (that is, genetically programmed) to take on the form of a required cell type and supposedly address a particular problem – a blank canvas in other words. In the case of PD patients, these stem-cells would need to be implanted to replace the damaged Dopamine-producing cells in the substantia nigra of the brain.

By the start of the 21st Century, scientific researchers from biology/chemistry backgrounds, in search of funding, were saturating the media with claims that stem-cells would be the panacea to almost every conceivable human problem. Like the elixirs of the 19th Century carpet-baggers, stem-cells, we were told, would be good for whatever ails you, from lumbago to ingrown toe-nails and warts. Step right up and hand over a few hundred million dollars in research funds and the stem-cell elixir is yours to behold – the *good statistics* were all wheeled out:

"...see how close we are to solving all of life's little problems – if only we had more research money...We're on the verge..."

My journey through two centuries of neuroscientific research reached the present day as a I waded through the series of extraordinary claims in relation to the application of stem-cells which appeared in the media – claims that had clearly been initially embellished by researchers in order to make them attractive as a concept to the media and to potential benefactors. These already inflated claims were again embellished by the media in order to make them attractive to the public and to provide a bullet and 15-second story for the evening news. By the time the public heard about stem-cells it appeared that anything was possible. And then the politicians got involved.

What could be more entertaining than watching politicians around the world squirm as they debated a subject, based upon third-hand knowledge, which appeared to be derived from exaggerated and distorted media reporting of garbled interpretations of embellished scientific claims? What could advance the cause of science further than a group of people vehemently arguing for or against the legislation of technologies which none of the proponents or opponents appeared to really understand:

"Stem-cell research is good (it cures cancer – great for mankind)."

"Genetic engineering research is bad (it creates two headed cows – horrible)."

"But aren't stem-cells and genetic engineering interrelated?"

"In that case stem-cell research is bad – we don't want people with cancer breeding two headed cows – or good – maybe we can cure cancer in two headed cows – that's got to be good - which answer will win the most votes? I can be passionate and committed about either one."

With all of all this passionate debate going on, it occurred to me that, at least in the context of the neurosciences, the application of stem-cell research to PD presented a sense of déjà vu. The idea of replacing damaged Dopamine producing cells in the substantia nigra of the brain with all-new-and-improved ones was remarkably similar to the 1950s idea of replacing missing Dopamine with the then all-new-and-improved laboratory produced Levodopa. In both cases, two fundamental research questions had not been addressed:

- What caused the Dopamine producing cells in the brain to die off in the first place?

- Given that the stable (natural) state of a Parkinsonian brain was Dopamine-depleted, how would the brain react to the introduction of an artificial mechanism which increased the level?

In the 1950s and 1960s, researchers did not have the luxury of asking these two questions because people with PD were suffering from appalling symptoms that an ingested form of Levodopa appeared to significantly relieve – the issue of *why* the relief occurred was of secondary importance. But, half a century later, the basic questions remained – only the technologies that were proposed to address them had in fact changed.

The human brain is responsible for innumerable control loops which are used to regulate the functioning of the body and stabilize basic parameters (for example, core body temperature). In the brain, just as in many other facets of nature, control mechanisms are built in to maintain the status quo. Many of the control loops that perform these functions are also interdependent – that is, if we change one control loop by artificially disturbing it in some way, then other control loops endeavor to compensate for the problem by ramping up or down their activities.

An example of this phenomenon would be if a human jumps into cold water and the artificial disturbance (i.e., the cold water) attempts to shift the body's stable temperature downwards. Various control loops (which compose the body's autonomic nervous system) react against the stimulus in order to maintain the core body temperature. For example, the breathing rate increases; skin pores are closed; muscles are activated (shivering) to increase heat generation, and so on. Similarly, if a human goes into a sauna, then the autonomic nervous system reacts against the temperature rise by opening skin pores to cause sweating, and to maintain the stable core temperature of the body. The various control loops all work in concert to maintain a stable temperature. If the operation of one control loop is varied then others endeavor to compensate by either working harder or scaling down their activities accordingly.

Not surprisingly, therefore, at least from an engineer's perspective, when humans ingest some form of artificial stimulant (i.e., a pharmaceutical) which acts to perturb the current, natural state of the body, then various control loops come into action to react against it. Neuroscientists soon learnt that it was altogether simplistic to expect that giving people an artificial form of Dopamine to replace the naturally occurring one would provide a complete solution to PD. So, while to a sufferer, the Parkinson's state may appear to be unnatural, at least in terms of the internal control systems within the brain, it is the natural (stable) state at a given time. Scientists discovered that artificially attempting to change this stable state caused all sorts of other control loops to come into action to compensate – hence the unsurprising phenomena of medication side effects and the idiosyncratic nature of medication performance.

What neuroscientists didn't know was what all the control loops did; how all the interdependent control loops in the brain functioned, and to what extent each loop interacted with other loops. In engineering, people tend to avoid interdependent control loops because they are very difficult to analyze – even when there are only a few. Imagine the problem that neuroscientists faced when they discovered that the brain was composed of countless interdependent control loops, and that they had managed to identify only a few of them. With this in mind, the addition of any artificial stimulus to the brain was difficult to analyze and predict, except in terms of its outward, clinically-observable effect.

In the case of PD, the addition of Levodopa caused a number of interesting changes to other control loops in the brain. In 1998, research published by Tamara Hershey *et al.* (in the *Proceedings of the National Academy of Sciences of the United States*), detailed the sorts of changes that took place as a result of long-term Levodopa usage. For one thing, Dopaminergic cells in the brain eventually started decreasing their production. For another, cells in a region of the brain, known as the globus pallidus, decreased the number of available Dopamine receptors. The net result of these interdependent control loops exercising their authority was that it was more difficult for the brain to control motor movements. People with Parkinson's therefore developed what was referred to as Dopamine induced Dyskinesia (DID) which was manifested in spasms, tics and muscle clenching. In some cases they also developed *Bradykinesia* which was a slowness in movement. The net effect was that people who used Levodopa for prolonged periods could have more dramatic transitions (as medication depleted from *on* to *off*) than new users because other control loops within the brain had made adjustments for the presence of the artificial stimulus (the ingested Levodopa).

What appeared, to medical researchers, to be an idiosyncratic effect of medication was, to an engineer, the blindingly obvious outcome of tinkering with a complex control system that one did not fully understand. Take a stable system – perturb that system in some small way – the net short term result is a shift from the status quo and a marginal change in performance – other interdependent control loops come into play to restore the status quo – more external stimulus is required to improve performance – other control loops react more harshly to restore the status quo - the system becomes less and less stable as it begins to oscillate from one state to another. Putting it another way, if you tease a dog long enough, it will bite back.

The *bite back* was documented in some of the neuroscience literature, where it was debated that the use of Levodopa could actually accelerate the progression of PD because of the sorts of effects that were taking place. It was speculated that the long-term ingestion of Levodopa was hastening the death of cells by working Dopaminergic cells to death.

Understanding how the innumerable, interdependent control loops react to an enormous range of stimuli is an intractable task. So, given the need for quality of life improvements in people with various disorders, researchers often follow the *do no harm* medical dictum on the assumption that if an improvement occurs, even if we don't fully understand it, the approach needs to be pursued. In fact, even without detailed understanding, reasonable outcomes may still be achieved because the control loops in question are the dominant ones and the impact of the others is insignificant. The problem with pursuing this *hypothesis-based* (or phenomenological) research is that although it may lead to incremental improvements, it is statistically unlikely to ever lead to a cure because it is a shotgun approach.

So, what could happen in the case of stem-cell research, and the concept of adding stem-cells to Parkinson's patients? What could happen if a brain, naturally depleted of Dopamine producing cells, is artificially disturbed from its natural state by the addition of new cells? Unless neuroscientists know what event, process or control loop caused the degradation of the original cells, then they have to assume that the outcome associated with stem-cells will be as idiosyncratic as the artificial addition of Dopamine. What will the various control loops in the brain do when new Dopamine-producing cells are added?

- Optimistically, the result could be that patients achieve a greater form of normality than they do with medication because the damaged cells are replaced and a *dominant* problem had been repaired.

- Pessimistically, the result could be that the implanted cells die off just like the original ones (because the original cause of cell death is unknown), or that other unidentified control loops attempt to compensate for the disturbance caused by the new cells and thereby create a new and more disturbing range of idiosyncratic effects.

Self evidently, these questions cannot be fully answered until the cause of PD is determined – and this is far easier said than done because of the slow progression of the disease – it can take months or years from the time that Dopamine producing cells begin to die off to the time when patients have noticeable symptoms – even then the symptoms can often be confused with other disorders.

One of my neuroscientific colleagues best summarized the prospects of applying stem-cells, in the absence of a complete understanding of the underlying causes of neurological disorders, thus:

"...it's like sprinkling iron filings over the top of an old Volkswagen and expecting it to turn into a new Porsche..."

So, in terms of PD, despite the fact that sufferers were desperate for a cure, expending time and resources on finding causes was important.

In essence, medical researchers tend to classify the causes of various diseases into a few main sources:

- Hereditary factors
- Lifestyle or physical incident
- Genetic mutations
- Toxin-based reactions
- Virus-based reactions.

If statistics and biological tests show that a particular disorder is clearly not hereditary then, without an enormous amount of research and experimentation, the other causes generally become an impressive sounding medical euphemism for *just one of those things*... It is very difficult to scientifically validate one of the other causes without an enormous number of independent epidemiological studies.

The *just one of those things* phenomenon takes the research problem back to one of serendipity – if researchers have access to a large cluster of patients who all contract a particular disease at a well defined point in time then there may be a slim chance of tracing the outbreak to some specific triggering phenomenon (e.g., a virus or toxin). If no single (time-limited) triggering phenomenon is found, then there needs to be an assumption that the disorder is the result of some ongoing occurrence – a natural deterioration or lifestyle-induced problem. Therefore, unless it turns out that PD is caused by a single-event, *big-bang*, then the addition of stem cells will have little impact because the artificially added ones will presumably die off just as the original ones did – because the same *undefined*, deterioration phenomenon is still present.

From time to time, clusters of various diseases do occur but the difficulty is in determining their statistical (that is, scientific) merit, rather than just the fact that they are interesting occurrences for their own sake. The media loves interesting cluster occurrences of diseases – scientists, however, need to treat them for what they are.

By way of example, consider that if a person took a camera to a busy city intersection and snapped a hundred photographs during the course of a day – a number of observations could be made. Firstly, and superficially, the people in the photographs might all appear normal and no inference would be made. Secondly, one could interview every individual in every photograph and ask them for their complete medical history – ten unrelated people in one photograph may all have cancer; five people in another photograph may all have had heart attacks; seven people in another might have renal problems, and so on. The only connection that these people may have is that they happen to be at the same intersection at the same instant in time.

One could say that the likelihood of having seven unrelated people with renal problems, in the same intersection at the same time, would be millions (or billions or trillions) to one against. But, such is the nature of statistics – if one took another billion (or trillion) photographs at the same intersection, one might not find another occurrence of seven people with renal problems. The fact that they all happen to be in the one photograph may be purely coincidental, or it may even be that there is no coincidence at all, and that the photographer merely happened to snap a picture of the *Renal Failure Walking Club* on their daily constitutional.

In PD research, two often-cited historical cluster cases sparked significant research interest. The first was a viral outbreak in a group of people which led to a severe neuropsychiatric disorder that was Parkinsonian like and, after many years, ameliorated (for a short period) by treatment with Levodopa – this became the subject of a now famous book by Oliver Sachs and a subsequent movie called *Awakenings*. The second was the onset of severe Parkinsonian symptoms in people who had ingested an artificially produced Heroin. These clusters led researchers to consider the *big bang* theory of PD, wherein it was speculated that a single event (virus or toxin) could have led to the onset of the disease in general – a quantum leap in reasoning from the relatively small numbers involved in the clusters but, nevertheless, still a good basis for further investigation.

The *big bang* theory of PD was particularly important to those researchers promulgating the notion of stem-cells as a cure for the disease. In particular, the idea of a single, time-limited trigger event was critical to their argument that replacing damaged cells had the potential to cure the disease – because the trigger event was no longer present to keep destroying newly implanted cells. Even with this optimistic scenario, the notion that this would lead to a complete cure was still unfounded, to the extent that it did not take into account how the brain would react to the introduction of a disturbance (i.e., the new cells) to the quiescent state of the Parkinsonian brain. In other words, the innumerable control loops within the brain of a PD person have already established a stable (albeit undesirable) control state which exists with a depleted number of Dopamine producing cells – what will they do if this state is disturbed by adding new cells? Will they revert to doing what they did in the pre-Parkinson's state? The answer is that scientists don't know because they don't understand enough about the brain. The corollary is that, if stem-cells do cure PD, they will probably do so long before scientists fully understand why.

If you are already overwhelmed by the scale of the scientific issues associated with curing a disease, consider the problem of selling research to the public when there are also political, business and economic concerns that influence scientific research directions. In particular, the political ones are often those related to public acceptance/resistance of/to any emerging technologies or therapies (e.g., stem-cells) and the business/economic ones being those that threaten sunk-investments in existing businesses or, indeed, large turnovers associated with existing technologies or therapies.

It is one thing to apply science to cure people of a disease but quite another to cure companies of their existing multi-billion dollar businesses.

For all the noise that scientists make about truth triumphing over vested business interests, the problem that scientists face is that truth is often very complex and multidimensional. Consider, for example, that in the 1950s scientists discovered the detrimental health effects of tobacco smoking and, half a century (and tens of thousands of person-years of scientific research) later, the tobacco and cigarette industries were as successful as they had ever been in selling their products – they just kept finding new markets as the Western markets depleted.

A victory of science (or truth) over vested business interests is predicated on two naive assumptions – one being that truth in science is simple and absolute, and the other being that big business is too dumb to hire their own eminent scientists to put forward contradictory and equally valid scenarios.

In some cases, the sheer magnitude of the financial pull of vested business interests is sufficient to also influence both the directions and benefits of science. For example, from a pure business perspective, it would not be unreasonable for organizations who develop a one-off, *silver bullet* cure for a disease to expect to be paid the same amount of money (or much more) for their cure than is paid for ongoing treatment. After all, if thirty years of medication for a Parkinson's patient is valued at, say, $100,000, then a valid business assumption might be that an organization proffering an immediate *silver bullet* cure (rather than treatment) deserves be paid, say, $1,000,000 for curing each patient – because they are providing a much better patient, economic and societal outcome. This sort of payment might be applied even if the real cost of the treatment, including amortization of research and development costs, is $20,000 per application.

Normally, pharmaceutical pricing is the product of negotiations between the manufacturer, governments and health insurance/maintenance providers. However, if, in the final analysis, a pharmaceutical company genuinely believes that neither governments nor health insurance/maintenance providers will be prepared to pay their preferred *silver bullet* prices, then why would they, in a business sense, vigorously pursue them in a research sense and risk losing a large percentage of their current business? The answer is that this would only occur if a competitor company was potentially able to release a cure and thereby neutralize a core business item. If the financial entry barrier for new pharmaceutical and therapeutic products was low, then the industry would, self-evidently, be more entrepreneurial and vigorous in its pursuit of new therapies because small, new players would always be a threat. The reality, however, is that the cost of getting such products into the global market is measured in hundreds of millions of dollars, which leaves the field dominated by large players who enjoy a stable income stream from conventional life-long-usage products.

Every now and then one would come across starry-eyed academic researchers proposing some new funding scheme or other which would supposedly assist hard-nosed biotechnology and pharmaceutical companies in moving things "out of the research arena" and into the commercial products arena. The naïve assumption was that by providing funding at the early business stages following research, risks would be mitigated and companies would be eager to move new therapies from the research laboratories to the supermarket shelf.

The unfortunate problem with the noble intentions of the researchers is that any cursory examination of how pharmaceutical companies derive income and profits indicates that real innovation is not a high priority. Although the word "innovation" appears frequently in pharmaceutical rhetoric and in marketing vocabulary, the reality is that business is derived from "cranking the handle" on conventional long-term treatments. When terms such as "innovative" or "revolutionary" appear, they often refer to minor modifications to old treatments that have enabled companies to maintain some form of licensing over their product. Hence, in the PD area, patients were generally exposed to innumerable "Dopamine Agonists" that were touted as being revolutionary new treatments.

The distortion of research and scientific benefits is further compounded because the patenting and licensing of technologies, particularly biotechnologies, has become a complex issue in its own right. In the late 20th Century, there was an enormous push to patent every uncovered permutation of DNA, with some expectation that this would yield massive financial rewards in the future. The ramifications of this were also significant in a research sense because they had the potential to either severely restrict the sort of research that could be undertaken, or to increase the cost of medical research, because of the need to pay royalties even for experimentation with various genetic materials.

So, now you have some inkling of the scientific, business and political factors at play. But, in case you aren't already overwhelmed by all these issues, consider now the answer to the simple question which relates to the researchers themselves:

What is the "truth" of the state of science or research in a particular field at a particular point in time?

To those outside the research world, this may appear to be an odd question to ask – surely all researchers are honest, and the current (and true) state of human knowledge is embodied in countless research journals? Isn't that what the media tell us when they report a new medical finding that has been published in some prestigious medical journal? Unfortunately, this is the naïve view – it assumes that what is embodied in scientific and medical journals is both accurate and true. Neither of these assumptions are necessarily justified.

Research publications represent the claims of various researchers – not necessarily facts or truth. The claims need to be independently verified – and this is a complex and time consuming process.

For those outside the research arena, it needs to be understood that when researchers make a claim, in order to gain credibility, they need to submit the claim to an independent group for peer review. In many cases, this occurs by submitting a research paper to a journal. High quality journals have expert peers to assess each paper and the claims therein before they are printed. This, of itself, however, does not guarantee that what is printed is factual. If, for example, a clinical study is performed and documented in a research paper, peer reviewers for a journal have no real way of knowing whether results were incorrectly acquired, accurately reported or even deliberately falsified by the researchers. The best that they can do is to apply their expertise to see if the *reported* work appears to have been systematically conducted and documented in line with specialist knowledge in the field.

So, how do we ever know what the reality of scientific research is?

The answer to this question is really quite complex. In general, if one research group makes a scientific discovery, and then publishes their work in a refereed journal, then we have an initial layer of screening – a basic peer review process. The big test of reality (or truth) only comes when other researchers can reproduce the work elsewhere, or use it as the basis of other research. The more that independent groups assess and use a piece of work, and validate/reproduce the outcomes, the more likely it is that a piece of research represents the *truth*. This validation process may take years or even decades.

In the latter half of the 20th Century, bureaucrats decided that performance measures needed to be applied to research outcomes, and this had the net effect of making the search for truth in science much harder. A common form of performance/productivity measurement in universities and research organizations was to determine how many research papers had been published in a given year. Researchers, being humans, naturally moved to maximize the number of annual publications and their career prospects by publishing as much as possible. Often the research that slipped through the publication process was questionable. So, in simple terms, volume went up but proportional truth content went down.

To remedy this problem, research bureaucrats then determined that it was far better to measure research quality by measuring how many times a research paper had been read and cited by other researchers – this is referred to as the *citation rate* or the *impact* of a research paper. A research paper with a large number of citations is presumed to be *good*, or at least *valid*, because this means that other researchers have probably used and verified the results. The simplistic bureaucratic reasoning was that this would serve to increase volume and *truth*.

However, the bureaucrats didn't count on the fact that researchers were humans, and being humans they sought to maximize their citations by having colleagues cite their papers and by creating citation loops. You can probably see where all this is heading – no matter what numerical indicators the bureaucrats put in place to police the publication of *truth* in science, humans always found a way around them to maximize their career or financial opportunities.

There were consequences to what happened in terms of the attempts to measure research by simplistic numbers. The first was that a proportion of what was published as science was essentially noise (publication for the sake of publication) and it was therefore difficult to separate *truth* from noise. The second was that the only meaningful validation process that was available in science was time. That is, if published research was applied by many other researchers, and continued to be applied for year after year, then we assumed that the work had a significant impact and was probably important. So, if a medical researcher laid claim to curing a disease by publishing in a renowned international medical journal, then the scientific *truth* of that claim may not become clear for another decade. From a patient's perspective, however, this is not necessarily a major problem. In medical research, if a claimed treatment is perceived to be non-harmful, and potentially beneficial, then it still may make its way to sufferers through experimental/clinical trials, before the natural scientific validation takes place.

Returning to our example of research into PD, we can surmise that, after two centuries of research, the current state of progress and treatment has come about as a result of science, serendipity, coincidence, natural business development and commercialization, and the emergence of enabling technologies. At the time we commenced our little research project into the field, the political debate into stem-cells had only begun to influence research directions, and the effect of any economic threat to core pharmaceutical products had not yet surfaced at a public level.

As an example of the progression of one scientific field, over the centuries, the investigation of PD also highlights the difficulties faced by researchers in pursuit of funding. Would PD have been cured by providing greater funding for research in 1817? By increasing funding by a million-fold or a billion-fold? Most likely not. The enabling sciences and technologies were simply not available to facilitate a cure, regardless of the available funding. Would PD have been cured earlier as a result of enabling technologies alone? In the second half of the 20th Century, the enabling sciences and technologies exploded and yet there were no major breakthroughs in the treatment of the disease after the advent of Levodopa. The progress, in this area of research, such as it was, came about as a result of the convergence of a complex combination of factors.

We then also need to consider the obvious follow up question – at what point do scientists know enough about any problem to categorically state that an increase in research funding will lead to a solution within a year or a decade or a century? The answer is that, until scientists know how many starting points there are to a problem; how many steps there are along each path; how many paths need to be explored, and how much time each path takes to explore, then they cannot predict, with any degree of certainty, the length of their mission. What is more, with many complex problems, scientists cannot even speculate on the number of starting points to the resolution of the problem. In retrospect, 19th Century research speculation on the potential starting points for a remedy to PD may appear extraordinarily naïve or even silly – but this is with a hindsight based upon almost two centuries of technological and scientific development that facilitated the current thoughts on the subject. With the benefit of another century of technology and scientific development, it may be that today's insight into how the problem could be tackled will, again, appear naive.

The other lesson to learn here is that it is not simply a case of two centuries of research into PD that has facilitated the current thinking into the disease – it is two centuries of research into areas such as quantum physics and semiconductor physics; the development of the microprocessor and supercomputer; advanced software systems; genetic engineering; advanced imaging equipment based on theoretical and applied physics; diagnostic testing and tools; the development and simulation of pharmaceuticals, and pharmaceutical manufacturing, and so on. With this in mind, if we again go back to 1817, and consider the consequences of focusing funding and efforts entirely on PD research, to the exclusion of other areas of science and technology, then it is evident that little progress would likely have been made, despite the resources consumed.

The problem with all of these issues is that they are not something that scientific researchers like to talk about in public. After all, why would they? Basically, the sheer weight of numbers tells us that, in many cases, the cure for an ailment, within the space of one human lifetime, has a significant element of serendipity, and stumbling across the right path, early on in the investigative process. Fortunately for the researchers, the mass media doesn't appear to understand these figures either, so they seldom get mentioned in public. And, they certainly don't appear in the marketing literature pertaining to research. After all, from a marketing perspective, it doesn't sound terribly encouraging for a researcher to tell prospective benefactors that, in scientific terms, and in the worst case scenario, a donation of a hundred thousand dollars will reduce the time taken to cure a disease from one billion years to 999,999,998 years.

Many novice researchers are also shielded from the harsh reality of research, which is that the overwhelming number of them will spend their entire lives simply following dead-end pathways and crossing them off the list of potential options. From the hundreds upon hundreds of thousands of researchers that carry out research in various fields, perhaps a few dozen, in the course of an entire century, will strike the mother lode (the correct path) with their work.

The other side of the equation also has to be considered, however. The simple fact of the matter is that regardless of the surrounding political and economic issues, without research, societal progress comes to a halt. The ongoing technological and scientific development of a society leads to all sorts of enabling technologies and an increasing knowledge base that can more efficiently eliminate potential starting points for the resolution of problems such as diseases – thereby reducing the time taken, from a billion years to, say, a hundred years or even ten years.

In the case of PD, and our small research project, what all the tens of thousands of pages of research papers didn't convey was the very personal issue of how difficult it was for people to cope with the disease itself. Certainly the research talked about symptoms and mobility measurement tests, and mobility scores, and so on. These were a convenient tool for classifying experimental subjects but they didn't really give an insight into the extraordinarily idiosyncratic nature of the disease and to the tribulations which it caused. Tribulations which, of themselves, might have been minor to a researcher or medical practitioner but which, to a sufferer, made every day frustrating and unpredictable to the point of severely eroding basic quality of life and the enjoyment of life. So, were the scientific researchers really *on the verge* of a cure to this insidious problem?

Cures in science tend to come either from detailed understanding or from serendipity. Better treatments, however, can sometimes arise from hypothesis based research. In the neurosciences, understanding had evolved significantly from its 19th Century beginnings but it was far from being a detailed understanding of how the brain worked, and why it sometimes didn't. Hypothesis-based research in the field was plentiful and yielding small but ongoing improvements for disease treatment, largely based upon pharmaceutical products.

As for serendipity – if Sister Kevin was around, she would probably have told us that far away cows have long horns.

6 WHAT HAPPENED NEXT

At this point, you are probably expecting that you have reached the part of the book where you are entitled to hear about some revelation that miraculously came to us in regard to Parkinson's Disease (PD) and its cure – the *Lorenzo's Oil*, the *Flux Capacitor*, the *banana and bag of peanuts cure* or, perhaps – for the Gilligan's Island fans, even the curative properties of *Mary-Anne and Ginger's coconut cream pie*. In the 1960s sci-fi movies all they ever had to do was to *reverse the polarity* of something in order to fix almost any catastrophic problem. Unfortunately, no such thing here. As far as this story is concerned, we have only gotten up to the part where we had to go and recruit participants for our research project.

In a medical research institute, the task of recruiting participants for an experimental research study would generally be a straightforward one that would be left to the devices of a postgraduate research student, or even an administrative person with specific duties in this area. This is a reasonable course of action because the researchers in such institutes are often people who already have medical degrees, and they are surrounded by other people who also have medical degrees. Our institute, however, was neither a medical research institute nor a neuroscientific research institute. It was an industrial research institute and the bulk of our staff were engineers – so too were the bulk of our research students. Our patients were cars, machine tools, lasers, computers and biomedical devices – none of these had ever complained about our bedside manner, or about the way in which we treated them.

As an institute, we were somewhat uncomfortable with the way in which we would handle the recruitment process for a study that would involve humans rather than machines, and so it was decided that I should go out to do the recruitment rather than our postgraduate researcher. This was the first of many *seemed like a good idea at the time* ideas that we had. What we didn't really consider was the fact that sending engineers out to deal with humans was probably not a good idea even at the very best of times.

The other *seemed like a really good idea at the time* idea that we had was for me to fulfill our commitment to go and visit a young-onset PD group meeting to recruit for volunteers. This could technically only go ahead in our university if the human research ethics committee had given prior approval to the proposed series of experiments that we had in mind.

As it turned out, the next meeting of the young-onset PD group was to take place before we would officially have formal notification of the status of our research ethics application. The advice we had was that it would be inappropriate for me to discuss the proposed project with the PD group, without ethics approval, because the university was not officially conducting or condoning such research until such approval was given.

In as much as the young-onset group only met quarterly, missing a meeting would delay participant recruitment for our project by three months. So, after discussions with the ethics people, it was agreed that I could attend the meeting and tell the group that there was an impending project, subject to ethics approval, and to ask for people who were interested to keep this in mind. To make matters more difficult, we were not even permitted to collect the names and contact details of interested people, because we didn't have ethics approval to do so. The strategy, therefore, would be to contact the group, after ethics approval had been granted, and let the group advise its members.

All of this seemed simple enough, so I got in touch with the person that coordinated the young-onset group to ask if I could attend the upcoming meeting, just to let people know that we would be looking for their assistance in the near future. The coordinator told me that this would be fine and, on the assumption that all I would have to do was a five-minute presentation, I decided (that is to say, it *seemed like a really good idea at the time*) that there was really nothing for which to prepare. However, as it turned out, this probably wasn't the best possible strategy.

Upon arriving at the young-onset group meeting, I discovered that the coordinator, with which I had been liaising, was not going to be present and had been replaced by another lady, whom I assumed to be some form of nurse.

Now, I have already told you that allowing engineers to interact with humans is probably risky enough at the best of times, but allowing engineers to interact with medical people is probably even worse. Engineers and medicos have completely different mindsets, and we often don't get along terribly well. Add to this mix the intrinsic sarcasm of the engineer, and the intrinsic piety and arrogance of the medico, and the resulting formula is highly flammable.

Speaking on behalf of the engineers, if we had to nominate the one characteristic of the medicos that annoys us more than any other, then we would nominate their condescending, *all-knowing*, medical mannerism – more specifically, the way in which they seem to treat those who don't happen to be other medical people. The basic medico premise appears to be that those from a non-medical background are deaf, stupid and completely incapable of understanding speech at a normal level and speed.

For engineers, condescending speech patterns are enough to push all of our buttons, including the all-important *Enter* key. So, when the person in charge of the PD session (who was probably a very nice lady) politely and innocently asked me, in her slow, loud medico voice,

"WOULD YOU LIKE A CUP OF TEA OR

COFFEE BEFORE WE START DARLING?"

all my engineering buttons were pushed, and my engineering sarcasm was activated,

"N O. T H A N K Y O U," I replied in the same slow, loud patronizing tone. This *seemed like a really good idea at the time* but, in retrospect, was probably not. It did, however, succeed in alienating me in record time, even for an engineer, and in earning me a dagger-eyed glare which I was able to translate into a vote of no confidence.

In looking around the room, it became apparent that even though the people present were part of a young-onset PD group, many of them were not actually young per se, and had been members of the group for more than ten years. In fact, the average age of the group was somewhere in the mid-50s. The other thing that became apparent was that some of the people in this group appeared to have very severe symptoms, with a few displaying the sort of dyskinesia that is often associated with long term usage of the L-Dopa drug. And, one assumed that these people were all in the *on* state of their medication – that is, their medication was fully ingested and they were as functional as they could possibly be given the current progression of their PD.

The meeting went through its initial formalities and then I was introduced to the audience – not as someone who was just going to briefly mention an upcoming research program but, rather, as someone who had come specifically to give a lecture on PD and the *advanced* research that we were currently undertaking.

I could hardly believe my ears as I listened to the introduction. Was this the retribution for my earlier *seemed like a really good idea at the time* remark? I wondered.

The dyskinetic movements of the young-onset group would have paled into insignificance compared to the apoplectic state of a university research ethics committee if they heard that I was conducting a lecture on a medical area completely outside my realm of expertise, and talking about a research project that had not even been considered, much less sanctioned. I stood up fairly slowly trying to think of what on earth I was going to say.

Obviously, even if I knew enough about the subject, it wasn't for me to give such a lecture, and nor could I now say that I had no intention of giving a lecture – and contradict the convener in front of the meeting. I decided that I might just as well try the truth as a first alternative– it seemed as good an option as any other, and besides, there really wasn't sufficient time to come up with a half-way decent lie.

I decided to begin by telling the group that I was really there as an imposter, and that I was a doctor of engineering not medicine. It was difficult to tell from the stunned silence whether the stone-faced audience reaction was the result of their Parkinsonian affliction or just the normal *Easter Island Syndrome* that people usually have when we tell them that we are engineers.

I decided to press on by telling the group that the issue I wanted to raise was about a project that was being conducted by someone who was a candidate in a doctor of philosophy program. I then gave them my usual definition of a doctor of philosophy in order to explain what was going on – that is,

"Someone who endeavors to learn almost everything about next to nothing so that they can get a job where they pretend to know everything about everything until they eventually realize that they know almost nothing about anything."

I was quite pleased with my opening which earned a good laugh from the group and another glare from the convener. The nurse had clearly come from the *diseases are meant to be serious* school of medicine, to which I had great difficulty in relating. Not surprisingly, the engineering world has long recognized that medicos, in general, have no sense of humor and, at this session, I had apparently hit the mother-lode.

Our engineering conclusion is that while we engineers are having our sarcasm machinery installed in the hospital birthing room, the medicos are being equipped with pious-assertiveness. Of course, in fairness to the medicos, the difficulty that they face in professional life is that if they don't appear forceful, decisive and completely incontrovertible, then patients may elect not to follow their advice or procedures. Worse still, patients might actually ask the blindingly obvious question of *"why?"* a few times, thereby leading them to the conclusion that the medicos don't know anywhere near as much as their veneer of confidence suggests.

The challenge for engineers in dealing with medicos is to get them to admit that they don't know as much as they claim. The key to this is to always ask lots of difficult and embarrassing questions, until the medicos crack and admit that they don't know. The first question that has to be asked by any engineer is,

"Why?"

which is followed up with,

"Do you have scientific evidence for that, or is this just your personal opinion?"

If neither of these succeed, then a confidence breaker question needs to be brought into play,

"And what do you think would happen if I decided to completely ignore your advice, given that it appears to be subjective anyway?"

followed by,

"Can you recommend any other doctors in the field who are more knowledgeable and can give me a more-informed opinion?"

Eventually, the medicos run out of fire power, admit that they don't know as much as their bravado suggests, and it is then possible to carry out a normal conversation – or at least normal for an engineer.

The idea of baiting medicos with questions always struck me as being a good one, from the perspective that I was always going to be the *baiter* rather than the *baitee*. In showing up to this meeting, therefore, the thought had never even crossed my mind that I was the one who was now going to be the *baitee* – the hunter had suddenly become the hunted. In retrospect, it shouldn't really have been a surprise that this was the case, because people with PD had had to learn to live with an extremely frustrating and demoralizing disorder. Obviously they had been told, just once too often, by one too many experts, about what was good for them. So, had I considered all this earlier, I might have realized that they were going to question anything and everything that I told them. And, they did.

Whenever I lectured to undergraduate engineers, I always told them that there were no such things as stupid questions – just stupid people who asked them and didn't deserve to pass the subject. Normally, this was enough to kill off any embarrassing questions (such as *why?*) for the rest of the subject. Obviously, this tactic wasn't going to work here.

In order to get the ball rolling, I began by summarizing what we proposed to do in our little research program. It seemed to me that I had done a really good job in summarizing the situation, and the reasons that we had for looking at the auditory brainstem response (evoked response) of people with PD. And then the questions started:

"Why are you just looking at evoked auditory response? Why aren't you looking at the evoked visual response as well?"

"Have you read the paper by X who did a study on evoked visual response?"

"Why don't you measure evoked auditory response over an entire day –

why do you just want to take measurements three times?"

"Have you considered X...?"

"Have you thought about Y...?"

And, so it went, for a good 20 minutes. The outcome was gradually becoming clear to me – it was going to be what we engineers referred to as a CFD outcome. CFD is an acronym that we engineers sometimes use for *computational fluid dynamics* and, more frequently, for *complete fucking disaster*. In this case, it was the latter definition that sprang to mind. And, just as things appeared as though they couldn't get any worse, I decided to tell the group about the ethics procedures associated with the research, which also *seemed like a really good idea at the time.*

"We would ideally like to have you come in for an entire day for testing but this is only an exploratory study, so we can't really get ethics approval for something that would be so intrusive," I told them.

"Well that's just plain crap!" said one of the audience.

"If we want to volunteer our time to doing a study for a day, then that's nothing to do with your ethics committee," said another.

By this stage, I could sense the room spinning around me as the noise level started to escalate with background sounds of,

"Here here," and, "That's right – it's nothing to do with other people – we can volunteer for whatever we like – it's our business."

I made another attempt at explaining the situation,

"I accept that it is your decision if you want to volunteer for something, and that research ethics committees have no control over that. They do, however, have control over what I can ask you to volunteer for, and this is based on the potential societal benefits weighed up against any risk or inconvenience to you. The procedures are there to protect your interests."

"We don't need other people to protect our interests – we're quite capable of making our own decisions."

"Well you might be capable of making your own decisions but, on this matter, I can't. I am bound by ethics procedures of the university and those procedures are tied up in government legislation. If I was to breach those basic guidelines, both I and the university could get into serious trouble. The issue here is that the people who write ethics procedures understand that many people, such as yourselves, are willing to offer their time and services to assist in research. The idea of the ethics procedures is to prevent researchers from unreasonably preying on the goodwill of people who want to volunteer, by using them for research which is not independently assessed to be of value to society."

I thought that this was a great winning argument which I had forcefully put forward. Needless to say, it received a rapturous response,

"That's just complete and utter bureaucratic bullshit!"

"Well, that's as may be, but it's government-legislated bureaucratic bullshit and, whether you accept it or not, our current research is only exploratory and what we would be asking you good people to do is to come to have your auditory response tested three times – once in the morning, soon after your medication; once in the afternoon, just before your medication, then a half hour or so after you take your afternoon medication."

And, just as I thought that I couldn't possibly look any sillier, then came the fateful comments:

"Afternoon medication? What afternoon medication? I don't think you understand," said one.

"No, I don't think he understands at all," said another.

And then, the pièce de résistance:

"And just how often do you think that I take my medication?" asked another person in the audience.

Interestingly, when I had looked round the room on entering the meeting, this was the one person that I had visually singled out as having been the least affected by the disease – during the meeting there were no severe tremors or dyskinesia. Needless to say, however, from the tone of the question, I just knew that no matter what I said, it was going to be the wrong answer. It was clearly one of those,

"...*and just how old do you think I look?*"

questions to which there is never a correct answer. So, as I ventured down the gangplank of the Titanic, I could already sense the impending aroma of iceberg,

"Three times?" I queried, while grimacing in anticipation of the response.

"I take my medication every half an hour – every half an hour – what would you suggest that I do if I want to come in for the tests?"

I was somewhat taken aback by the significance of what this person had just said, and its implications. This was a life that literally had to be tied to a digital clock for almost every waking moment as a result of their PD. No sooner had one dose of medication been taken than this person had to start preparing for the next dose. As I felt myself dissolving into the floor at this response, I could feel the room revolving around me with a cacophony of other similar questions and comments:

"Sometimes I take my medication five times a day but I vary it on different days."

"I take mine three times but I have the last two doses later in the evening so I am not as stiff when I get up in the morning."

"I take my medication at all different times, depending on how I feel and whether I sense the current dose wearing off."

"How are we supposed to get down to the university?"

Finally a question that I could answer. I responded with,

"We'll provide you with parking spaces and cover the cost of your car expenses."

However, this only served to dig a deeper hole for myself and, at this point, the convener of the session interrupted with,

"I think you had better consult with a neurologist before going much further. Most of these people are not able to drive."

"Well their carers can drive can't they?"

"Darling, you can hardly expect people's carers to spend hours driving them backwards and forwards for your research. And they can't use public transport. You need to provide them with taxis."

"Fine, I'll have our administrative staff mail them *cab-charge* vouchers before they come in – that's not a major problem."

"I think you should still consult with a neurologist first, anyway."

"Well, we already have a medical adviser with expertise in neuroscience."

"That's hardly a neurologist, darling."

"I know what a neurologist is. But, if it makes you happy, we'll engage a neurologist as a consultant before we start testing."

I was on the verge of ending my response to the nurse with *darling* or *sweetheart* but figured that the hole I had dug myself was probably already deep enough. Fortunately, the moment was interrupted by one of the audience asking,

"Why should we volunteer to do this for you anyway?" which was quickly responded to by someone else with,

"Well for the sheer fun of it all, I guess. It's been a barrel of laughs so far."

Just as I had convinced myself that this whole meeting had gone far worse than anything I had imaged beforehand, I bade the group goodbye and said that we would let them know closer to the time. However, as I left the meeting, one of the elderly members of the group came out behind me in his walking frame and said,

"Don't worry son, I'll volunteer – you can count me in."

This made me feel a little better about it – at least I had a sample size of one, which was one better than nothing. When I returned to the university, looking more than a little flustered, someone sarcastically asked me how the session went and I told them,

"Could have been worse."

"Do you think you'll get many volunteers soon?"

"As soon as hell freezes over is my early estimate."

"Have you succeeded in using your usual charm to alienate the entire Parkinson's community yet?"

"I haven't met all of them yet. I've only managed to alienate the ones that I've met. Which, if you think about it, is probably better than my average with the rest of the population."

The problem as I saw it was relatively simple. We engineers are actually very good at communicating with other engineers, and of course with cars, computers, remote controls, cordless telephones, power tools and other important elements of life as we know it – it's really only other humans that we have any problems with. You see, as I told you early on in this book, we engineers communicate with each other through poisonous and sarcastic barbs and, to paraphrase *Professor Henry Higgins* of *My Fair Lady* fame, it isn't really a question of how badly we treat someone but, rather, whether anyone has ever seen us treat anybody else better.

In retrospect, in regard to the young-onset group, I may have made a few teensy-weensy errors in my visit, and offending the nurse in charge had probably been the least of them. It also occurred to me that I had gone down to the session planning to talk to *people with Parkinson's*. That's what they called themselves, and even that had me unhinged from the beginning. Over the decades, the spin doctors had been working overtime to try and make diseases sound as pleasant and cheerful as possible. Since the time I was in Sister Kevin's class, *handicapped people* had become *disabled people*, and *disabled people* had become *challenged people* – as though the pleasant and cheerful nomenclature actually made as much as a razoo of difference to the people who had the problem.

People were no longer lazy but *motivationally challenged*. Humans were never fat but they could be *circumferentially disabled*. Short people were *vertically handicapped*, and tall people were *altitudinally challenged*. Interestingly, despite all the spin-doctors on the planet, people with PD referred to themselves as *people with Parkinson's Disease* which I thought, at the very least, exhibited a degree of dignity. Even so, I still had a problem with this collectivization of diseases because, fundamentally, it seemed to differentiate these people from the rest of the community – after all, people who sneeze aren't referred to as *people who sneeze*, and people with back pain aren't referred to as *people with back pain* – as though they are any different to anyone else. We tend to think of all these as just being people.

For the first time in my life, however, I had had to address a group that had been classified as *people with something*, rather than just people. And, as I have already explained, we engineers have enough difficulty communicating with people in general, without the added difficulty of the *with something*. Add to this the fact that *people with something* might not appreciate the language of engineering sarcasm or, worse still, take offence at it, like the millions of *people without something*, and I had just cause to make a complete fool of myself.

In thinking about how the meeting went, it also occurred to me that I had always secretly hoped that *people with something* were somehow completely different to *people without something* – maybe that they were all tall, or all short, or all fat, or all hunch-backed. The theory was that if the *people with something* were indeed different to the *people without something*, then that meant that the *people without something* wouldn't ever get the *something*.

The most disturbing thing that I experienced in seeing this group of *people with Parkinson's* was that these people weren't all tall, or all short, or all fat, or all thin, or all young, or all old. Some were tall, some were short, some were younger and some were older – some warm and friendly, and some were rude and cantankerous. Even more disturbing was the fact that some of these people were doctors or economists or businessmen or police detectives, or even engineers, and some were as sarcastic as I was. And that was a critical point that they omitted from the books and research papers on the subject.

Medical books and medical research papers are written in a form that suggests that these disorders happen to *people* – the implication being that these *people* are actually *other people*, rather than doctors or medical researchers. But, of course, the *people* can be doctors and nurses and engineers and scientists and, in the mix of this group, it became blindingly obvious that this particular disorder could pretty much happen to anybody. And, for every one or two hundred people in society, that *anybody* was a *somebody*.

My encounter also led me to wonder whether any of the people who were in the young-onset PD group had ever previously thought that they would contract the disease themselves? Probably not a single one. They too had probably thought that this was a disease that only affected *other people*.

Putting the philosophizing to one side, the meeting with the young-onset group had left me with two problems – one being that I still had to get participants with PD, and the other being that I had to swallow my engineering pride and consult a neurologist for advice. In particular, I needed to find a neurologist that was prepared to devote an hour of his/her time to a project that was not related to a medical research institute. It was almost axiomatic that many of them would be unlikely to be interested in helping. So, I decided that rather than swallowing my engineering pride and groveling for assistance, I would just call a neurologist and offer to hire them as a consultant, at whatever fee they wished to bill us.

After contacting the local PD support group, I was given the names of some neurologists, one of whom was highly regarded in the area of PD diagnostics and, because I didn't know any others, I presumed that he would be as good as any.

I contacted the neurologist's receptionist; explained the entire saga, and offered to have myself, my research co-supervisor and our medical colleague come and visit him for an hour – making it clear that we would pay the neurologist for his time, and that we were not asking him for a favor. The receptionist said that she would not organize an appointment unless the neurologist had first spoken to us about the meeting, and that she would pass the message on to him. I thought this was somewhat arrogant but figured, what the hell, let's see what he says.

One day went passed with no response, then another and another, and then another. I rang back the receptionist who said she would pass on the message again – the neurologist, she said, was *a very busy man.* I told her that I was *a very busy man* also – I didn't mention the fact that my two, principal diary entries for the year had been *"change cat's flea collar"* and *"garbage day has moved to Tuesday"*. Another two days went past and still no response. I called the receptionist again and was shuffled about from one hospital department to another, only to be told that the neurologist had already called but I wasn't in.

"That is simply not true," I said, "there is no record of any incoming calls from him on my phone's call register."

"He has an unlisted number, so it probably wouldn't show up," she replied.

"Then it would have appeared on my call register as an unlisted number calling, wouldn't it? And I don't have any record of any unlisted numbers coming in either – wonderful things these call registers aren't they?"

After a long pause, the receptionist responded with,

"And what is it that you wanted to discuss with him?"

By this stage, I was frothing at the mouth at what I perceived to be the arrogance of all of this, and I no longer had any interest in whether he was going to call back or not – I'd already made up my mind to find someone else. But, I just couldn't resist letting the receptionist have a taste of the cold steel blade of engineering sarcasm,

"It's about my having a brain hemorrhage. My lawyer says that if he has any decency whatsoever he'll get off the golf course and give me a call within the next ten minutes. Thank you for all your help. All the best."

I hung up the phone down and counted backwards,

"Ten. Nine. Eight. Seven. Six…"

Ring. Ring.

"Doctor, what a delightful surprise that you've chosen to return my call so quickly – you needn't have gone to so much trouble. It really wasn't all that urgent."

The rather breathless neurologist was clearly more than a little annoyed with having to provide an urgent reply, but I didn't particularly care. I got the result that I wanted, and obviously he also felt a little guilty about not responding for so long. I never did find out whether his receptionist had decoded the engineering sarcasm in my message and passed it on, or whether she had just told him that some deranged psychopath had called, desperately in need of some form of medication – I certainly wasn't game to ask.

Amazingly, rather than complaining, the neurologist actually commenced the dialogue by apologizing to me for the run around that I had been given. I explained that we wanted to hire him as a consultant for an hour or so to get information on our proposed course of experimentation. It turned out that I had had the guy all wrong – he was actually an extremely nice person,

"Don't be silly, you don't have to pay me. If it's research I'm happy to do whatever I can."

Even more amazing was the fact that he wouldn't hear of us wasting time to go and visit him at his hospital clinic. He offered to come down and visit us at our research institute. A few days later, three of us met with him to discuss the tests that we had in mind. He started the formalities himself with the conditions of his advice.

"Please understand that I am not going to make any comments about the validity or worth of the sort of tests that you are planning to do. I am only going to make comments on the sort of testing procedure that you have in mind, and what you can expect in dealing with people when they are not on medication."

I interpreted this as being his polite way of telling us that we were completely wasting our time and his, and that we didn't have the faintest idea of what we were talking about – but then, I thought that I had already misjudged him once before, so perhaps it was just his turn of phrase. I decided to restore my engineering sarcasm machinery back to its holster for the time being.

I told the neurologist about my recent encounter with the young-onset group – not the embarrassing parts of course (we engineers would never give an inkling of any weakness or failure to our medical foes), just the parts about the severity of the group's symptoms. I also mentioned the person who took their medication half hourly.

"I know that group fairly well and I also know the person to whom you are referring. I think that they are probably not the appropriate group for your experiments. First of all, most of those people have severe manifestations of PD. If you bring them in here with their medication *off*, you may have difficulty in handling them without some form of experienced nursing staff – I don't think it's a good idea unless you have trained staff on hand. That person you described that takes the medication half hourly – that's one of the more extreme manifestations of the disease – probably only represents one in a thousand cases. You should really be looking for a group of people who are only mildly afflicted. Put an advertisement in the state based Parkinson's newsletter – you should easily get 10 – 20 participants. I'll also make people who come to my clinic aware of the project – you understand that I can't promote it for you – I can only draw their attention to the study."

We then moved on to the issue of bringing patients in at various times of the day, so that we could measure their auditory brainstem response in the morning when their medication was fully *on*; in the afternoon when their medication was *off*, and again in the afternoon when their medication was back *on* again.

"Why don't you just tell them to not to take their medication when you want them *off* – I would."

"Well that's easy for you to say – you can do that – you're a doctor of neurology – I'm a doctor of engineering. I can't prescribe changes to their medication without ethics approval."

"Well, how do you propose to know whether they are fully *on* or *off* unless you give them mobility tests? Does your doctoral researcher have training in clinical mobility testing?"

Since I only had a vague idea of what mobility testing was, I thought it was a good idea to just say no.

"Well, ok then. Have him come to my clinic for a couple of afternoons a week, for a few weeks, and we'll have him trained to do mobility testing on my patients – he can do the *Hoehn and Yahr* test and the *Webster's* test. That will give you an accepted number that will indicate the level of impairment, and you can use that to help you judge whether the medication is *on* or *off* when you do your tests. It will also help the student to get used to dealing with people at various stages of the disease."

"How much is it going to cost us to have our doctoral candidate trained in mobility testing?" I asked.

"What is it with you engineers and money? You always want to pay for everything. I was going to do it for nothing – it's my pleasure," he grinned. "But I can charge you if you want."

We then went on to issues of medication and misdiagnosis of the disease. I gave him the figure of 25% in the misdiagnosis rate, to which he appeared to take some offence.

"You probably got that figure from my research paper. That's an old figure and the situation has improved considerably in the last ten years – the misdiagnosis rate is probably less than 5% with improved clinical methods."

The issue of misdiagnosis in PD had been reported in all sorts of research papers. I was somewhat surprised that he would suggest that we got the figure out of *his* paper – after all, lots of other people had researched the same subject – why would we have read *his* paper in particular? What was so special about it?

After the meeting, I thought that I had better go and check up on this neurologist and find out who the hell he was, and what was so special about *his* paper on diagnosis of PD. I logged on to the library's *Web of Science* database to try and locate *his* research paper. It turned out that *his* paper had been cited a staggering 840 times – his other papers had also been very highly cited, thereby making him a seriously eminent person in the international field. Luckily then, my engineering sarcasm machinery had been holstered, and I hadn't made the caustic remark I was planning to make when he referred to *his* paper.

In reviewing the situation, the whole research project now resembled the *curate's egg* – good in parts. As it stood, on the negative side, we had a grand total of one participant with PD, who we were told to exclude because he had a serious manifestation. That left us with a grand total of none. On the positive side, we had a professional neurologist to help us with mobility training, so that in the unlikely event that we ever did find a participant, we could assess their mobility. At least that was one far away cow in the hand, which was worth at least two in the bush – or wherever pairs of cows reside.

7 A TESTING TIME

You have now reached the part of the story where most of the work was conducted by our doctoral research candidate. Since my involvement with this part was very small, this means that I could either leave the next 20 pages of this book blank for you to make notes upon, or else just exaggerate the importance of my contribution. I have decided to choose the latter course of action. Not just for the purposes of self-aggrandizement, although you might accuse me of this anyway, but so that you can have a better understanding of what we were actually doing.

The first thing that I need to tell you is that our consulting neurologist, who didn't actually charge us a consulting fee, was true to his word and took our doctoral research candidate on as an apprentice for a few weeks so that he could be trained in the clinical assessment of Parkinsonian symptoms.

The clinical testing for Parkinson's Disease (PD) is somewhat interesting in its own right. In the late 1960s, when one of the key PD medication regimes (Levodopa) moved into common usage, people also began developing a range of tests that could be used to assess the level of impairment arising from the disease. These straightforward clinical tests provided a subjective (but, nevertheless, semi-standardized) way of comparing patients. One of these tests, developed in 1967 by Margaret Hoehn, became known as the *Hoehn and Yahr Staging Test*. This basically divided the disease into five distinct stages of progression. Each stage was characterized by a particular group of symptoms, and clinicians would endeavor to classify their patients as follows:

- *Stage 1* was where patients had mild symptoms on one side only, typically a tremor in one limb. Their posture may have changed and they may have noticed difficulty in realizing even simple facial expressions.

- *Stage 2* was where patients still had mild symptoms and minimal disability but their posture and gait were affected. At this stage, the disease had become bilateral (i.e., spread to both sides).

- *Stage 3* was where the disease progression had become quite debilitating and patients experienced a slowing in their body movements. Their equilibrium was affected and their ability to walk or even just stand up had noticeably deteriorated. Stage 3 sufferers could, however, still live alone with a degree of independence.

- *Stage 4* was where patients had severe symptoms that largely removed their independence. They could still walk but experienced rigidity and a marked slowness in movement (Bradykinesia). Such patients could not function alone and required a carer. Ironically, tremor in Stage 4 patients was sometimes less than in Stages 1 to 3.

- *Stage 5* was referred to as a *cachectic* stage. *Cachexia* is medical gobbledy-gook that describes people with chronic diseases who have reached a stage of muscle wastage, weight loss and general deterioration. In people with PD, this referred to the stage where afflicted people could no longer walk or stand and were defined as complete invalids. At this stage, sufferers generally required constant nursing care.

Many outsiders tended to view PD as being an affliction of simple tremors, leading to inconvenience or annoyance. However, the *Hoehn and Yahr* classification showed how comprehensively debilitating the disease could become. At *Stage 5*, PD also became life-threatening for a number of reasons. Firstly, there were the fundamental degradations of the immune, respiratory and circulatory systems in patients who had become immobile or bed-ridden. Many of these problems could rapidly become life-threatening and included bed-sores, urinary tract infections, digestive problems, pneumonia, gangrene, and so on. Secondly, in terms of the PD itself, patients could deteriorate to a stage where even swallowing was impractical, and they had to be *tube-fed*.

People therefore didn't necessarily die from PD per se but, rather, from all of the complications that arose in *Stage 5,* and their generally weakened state – often with such problems as pneumonia or various infections.

Of course, the staging tests didn't really do diddly-squat for a person with PD but they did give neurologists a sense of satisfaction in knowing that they had divided a disease into convenient pieces so that they could compare notes at medical conferences. It also helped in classifying the level of care and support that sufferers would require.

In terms of more directly assessing a patient's current status and the effectiveness of their medication, a range of mobility tests were also developed in the 1960s. One of these was a test, developed by D.D. Webster, and became known as the *Webster Rating Scale.* This was a series of simple tests that assessed the parameters of common human movement – that is, balance; gait; rigidity; ability to make facial expressions, and so on. For each parameter that was tested, a score was given. The higher the score, the higher the impairment. So, after having completed all the Webster tests, a person with PD would be given an overall score (by a clinician) which would numerically describe their mobility.

You may well ask why we actually needed to measure mobility in our research? Didn't PD just get worse the longer that people had it? Ironically, the answer to this question was no – this is part of the idiosyncratic nature of the disease. Some people that we encountered had had the disease for ten years or more and were still only mildly afflicted by it in terms of mobility. Some people who had had the disease for only a few years were severely disabled by it. Neurologists generally gave their patients *typical scenarios* for what would happen to them as their disease progressed but, by and large, when it came to PD, few people appeared to be text-book typical.

The important thing about mobility tests was that they provided a simple tool that enabled clinicians to determine how well a patient could cope at a particular point in time, or how effective a patient's medication was. As PD progressed, the value of the core medication (Levodopa) generally decreased and its long-term side effects increased. The transitions from medication *on* to *off* became far more pronounced and distressing. Modern ancillary pharmaceutical products could sometimes improve this situation by providing smoother transitions from medication *on* to *off*. In order to assess the general effectiveness of pharmaceutical treatments, standardized clinical mobility tests would be employed by pharmaceutical companies, neurologists and clinicians to get an objective measure of performance.

It was our consultant neurologist's view that the various staging and mobility tests were really just an aid to quantifying the sorts of characteristics that experienced neurologists could determine on a qualitative basis anyway. So, what our doctoral research candidate really needed was twenty years of neurological clinical experience condensed into three weeks of practice. This wasn't all that practical, given that we planned to start testing within a few weeks, so the next best thing was to get a first-hand insight into the key factors that were thought to be of significance, by a person who actually already had decades of clinical experience in the assessment of PD.

Now, just in case you have already forgotten what it was that we intended to do with our research, let me recap. This will help to fill up the twenty pages of the book that would otherwise have been blank.

Our intention was to measure the auditory brainstem response (ABR) of a group of people afflicted with PD and to compare a range of characteristics from this response against a control group – that is to say, a group of people with no history of neurological disorders. The people with PD were to be tested three times. Once in the morning (when they were fully medicated); once in the afternoon when they were almost unmedicated (i.e., just before they took their medication), and once an hour after they had taken their medication in the afternoon.

For the PD group, the testing procedure was quite onerous for two reasons. To begin with, participants had to come in to our institute at least twice because they couldn't just be expected to sit around from the morning session until late in the afternoon. Secondly, each time the PD people came in, they had to have a number of tests performed. For each participant, his/her temperature had to be measured, then their mobility assessed (through the Webster's test), and then he/she had an ABR recorded by stimulating each ear with a series of *clicking* sounds. All of this took close to an hour of each person's time at each session. The control group, on the other hand, had an easier time – all they had to do was to come in on one occasion and have their temperature and ABR recorded.

The reason that we had to record a person's temperature each time we measured their ABR was because earlier research by others had shown that the ABR could vary with core body temperature, and we had to know whether any changes were as a result of thermal irregularities from common causes (e.g., a viral infection) or the PD.

Years ago, recording body temperature might have been as straightforward as sticking a thermometer under someone's tongue (or into some other bodily orifice) but, in the modern world of medical ethics and its application to engineers interacting with humans, we needed to use a less invasive method. We decided to use a hospital-grade *tympanic* thermometer (that is, digital ear-probe), and it was my task to go down to the local pharmacy and acquire one for the project. A simple task, one might think.

Getting the thermometer was straightforward, and unwrapping it with all the joy and enthusiasm that any engineer would apply to a new technical toy was also easy. As I have already told you, we engineers feel that we have no need for instruction manuals, so the first step was just to apply the thermometer to my own ear to test its operation. This gave me a reading of zero degrees, indicating that I was either dead or that the thermometer was not functioning. As the obituaries had made no mention of my passing on that day, I assumed that the thermometer was, as we say in engineering parlance, *busted*.

Several other PhD qualified engineers came in and told me that I obviously wasn't using it correctly, so they all tried the same thing, and professionally concluded that the thermometer was probably *busted*. At this point, I decided to hand the thermometer over to my research student, who took it home and also concluded that it was *busted*. My research student then took the thermometer over to the sensory neurosciences laboratory whose staff also concluded that the thermometer was probably *busted*.

Up until this point, of course, nobody had broken the engineering code of ethics by actually reading the instruction manual. It was therefore left to me to make this transgression. The first page of the manual thanked me profusely for buying the thermometer and hoped that I would get many happy years of enjoyment out of this *precision instrument*. In fairness to the manufacturers, it was highly precise in the sense that it seemed to tell everyone that their temperature was exactly 0.00 degrees. With all else having failed, it fell upon me to return the device to the pharmacy and get a replacement.

"What seems to be the problem with it?" enquired the pharmacist.

"It's *busted* – it only ever reads zero degrees," I replied, with the level of technical detail that people come to expect from doctorally qualified engineers.

"We've never had one of these *busted* before – are you sure you're using it correctly?"

"Of course I'm using it properly, I have a PhD in engineering. Try it yourself."

After the pharmacist had tried it on himself and had come to the conclusion that he also had a "0.00" degree temperature, he concluded,

"You're right, it's *busted*. I'll order you a replacement."

The next day, the replacement arrived and we went through the whole process again. I even committed the mortal engineering sin of looking at the instruction manual for the second time. The conclusion – the thermometer was *busted*. So, back to the pharmacy.

As it happened, this time the pharmacist was taking a phone call when I arrived, so his assistant from the cosmetics counter asked if she could assist.

"Look, this is the second one of these digital thermometers I've bought here and it doesn't work."

"What seems to be the problem with it?"

"It's *busted*."

"Are you sure you're using it correctly?"

Now, this seemed to be a good point at which to turn on the engineering sarcasm machinery:

"Look, I don't want to be rude but I've got a PhD in engineering. I've tested it and it's *busted*. Our doctoral research student has tested it and thinks it's *busted*. Our sensory neurosciences people have tested it and they think it's *busted*."

At this point the pharmacist got off the phone and intervened with, "This seems very strange - let me try it," and again came to the same conclusion,

"It's *busted* alright. Still reads zero."

Unconvinced by the professional conclusions of a group of engineers with PhDs; our sensory neuroscience technicians, and the pharmacist himself, the cosmetics assistant persisted:

"Maybe you people just aren't using it properly. You need to hold your head straight, look forward and pull your ear-lobe back before you measure. You mustn't lean your head forward when you use it. Can I try?"

Just as I was in the process of telling the cosmetics lady that, in my professional *PhD-in-engineering-qualified* opinion, this was a complete waste of time, and hardly likely to make the slightest bit of difference to the outcome, she looked at the reading from the thermometer with a smile. I could hear a little voice inside me saying,

"Dear God, if there's any justice in the world for engineers, don't let this *Maybelline-eye-liner-expert* get a reading now after what I've said to her."

"See – works perfectly," she said, showing me the reading from the thermometer. "You just have to know how to use it properly."

As I did my now increasingly regular dissolves into the floor, I could hear her muttering something under her breath, along the lines of,

"PhD my aunt Fanny – why don't you try raising a couple of kids and see how much you learn…"

I was on the verge of making the comeback line,

"I don't have kids, lady. I have a PhD and I have cats. We're an evolved species – we don't need digital ear-probe thermometers."

But, alas, my ego was so dented that I was unable to activate my vocal chords. Why didn't I just throw the fucking thing out and go and buy another one from a different pharmacy – one without a cosmetics counter?

However, despite the humiliation involved in the acquisition process, it appeared that we now had a working thermometer. All we needed to continue our research were experimental participants.

When you have some position of authority in a research institute then control groups are easy to come by. A control group is what normal people would probably call *normal people*. You will note that we researchers don't call control groups *normal people* because they aren't necessarily *normal*. They're just people who don't happen to have (or at least don't think that they have) the disorder that we are comparing against. In our case our control group was made up of mostly engineers – you can judge for yourself, based on what I have already told you about engineers, whether you would consider these to be *normal* or not. Nevertheless, they were a control group and all we had to do to assemble them was to knock on office doors and ask people to go and volunteer to have their responses measured. So, this recruitment exercise only took a few minutes to complete and went far more smoothly than my earlier efforts with the young-onset PD group.

In terms of getting participants who were afflicted with PD, we ultimately decided to use a number of mechanisms, including the various Parkinson's newsletters, together with notices on the boards of movement disorder clinics. Interestingly, for a disease which had largely been shunned by the society around it, the people who did provide support were remarkably dedicated and committed and helped us enormously.

In applying the standard, pessimistic and shallow engineering approach to life, I simply made the assumption that nobody would ever bother volunteering because they were probably as shallow and cynical as I was. And, having seemingly gotten nowhere with the young-onset group, the rest of the recruitment process was probably going to be an uphill battle. Surprisingly, however, within a few days of the advertisements appearing, we started to get enquiries. Amazingly, people were actually going to volunteer.

My philosophy of making the best of smaller decisions and letting the bigger issues take care of themselves appeared to be working successfully again. In fact, if I had sent out a divine message, through a séance session with Sister Kevin, and gave her the ideal list of participant requirements for our study, we could not have gotten a better response than we did from the newsletter and notice-board advertisements.

In terms of our research, we were really interested in people who were only mildly afflicted with PD. There was little to be gained in diagnosing people who were already severely afflicted, because it was the diagnosis of the disease in its early stages that was important. We were interested in having a mixture of males and females to see if any of the results were gender biased. We were interested in having a range of age groups, from young participants in their late 30s and 40s to those in their 80s. We were interested in having people who had been diagnosed for various periods of time, from one to ten years. We were interested in having people who had a *deep brain stimulator* implant to see if this affected the results. Amazingly, with no planning or insight, somehow, we miraculously managed to get all of these factors in the first 15 volunteers who called.

I didn't do the mathematics but I'm sure that it would have statistically been far easier for a person to get hit by a bolt of lightning (or for an engineer to be a social success at a dinner party) than it would have been to get this particular mix of participants.

And, one by one, over the course of a couple of months, they started coming in to have their tests.

Every now and then, I had the opportunity of meeting some of the people while they were waiting to have their tests and just informally discussed their disorder with them. Not surprisingly, I suppose, the mature-onset participants were the ones who appeared to be coping best with the disease. Generally, they had an established support base in terms of their family; they were financially secure, in the sense that they didn't depend upon work to survive; and they were less concerned about the loss of mobility because it was largely expected from an age perspective anyway. The mature-onset people were also less self-conscious about how they appeared (i.e., in terms of tremors and dyskinesia, etc.) and more concerned with the fundamental issues of medication side effects and just getting through life.

As I have already told you, the most disturbing thing that I discovered about PD is that the people who get it appear to be so vastly different in makeup. Some are short, some are tall, some are young, some are old, some are thin, and some are fat. Some people are happy and outgoing, some are rude, cranky and introverted. Some people are edgy and in denial

– and some are totally accepting of the disorder and just see it as another part of life. Some are noble and some are self-centered. That is probably the part of the disease that I found most difficult to accept. It isn't really a fair disease – it hits nice people and nasty people just the same. I had secretly hoped that all of the people we had would turn out to either be all noble or all cantankerous or all fat or all thin. In my own engineering reasoning, I figured that if they all turned out to be nasty then I would change my life for the better and be nice – if they all turned out to be nice, I would become a complete prick (or, at least a bigger one than people have accused me of being). However, life and diseases clearly didn't work that way.

Some of the people that came in for testing, particularly a few of the elderly ones, were quite extraordinary people in their own right. One octogenarian had survived the Great Depression, the Second World War, and the Korean War – it was clear just from talking to him that he wasn't about to let something like PD get in the way of the rest of his life. After we had a telephone interview with him, we arranged for a time to have him come in, and our administrative staff mailed him taxi vouchers so that he could get to and from our building without any hassles. However, in the case of this old timer, he ended up arriving half an hour before his scheduled test. I asked him whether his taxi had arrived early. He responded,

"Didn't come by taxi. Didn't want to waste the university's money on a taxi fare, so I decided to walk. Here's your voucher back – you use the money for your research instead."

Interestingly, this *salt-of-the-earth* octogenarian, afflicted with PD, had actually just walked more than four kilometers, with a Zimmer walking frame, in order to participate in our test – and to save a university money. I tried to explain to him that this really wasn't necessary:

"Look, here's the deal. Universities waste more money in one day than you can earn in fifty lifetimes of work. So, the first rule in participating in research is never try to save universities money. Universities and research institutes all have lots of money. That's why we pay people huge sums of money to run these places, and go out into the public and tell them that we don't have any money – so that we can get more money to hire more people to tell the public that we don't have any money. So, what have we learnt here? The moral of this story is that you should keep the cab voucher we sent you and use it to visit your friends – you've earned it."

"No, I wouldn't feel right about that. I'll do you a deal instead. You take your voucher back and I'll think about coming here by taxi next time – unless it's a nice day, then I'll walk – and you can put the money to some good use."

So, having cut a deal on the taxis, we got onto discussing his PD and the novel way that he had found to deal with it and his medication:

"I went to one neurologist and he told me to take these," he said, removing one set of medication from his coat pocket, "and then another one told me to take those ones, and then I got another set. One lot of medication gave me diarrhea; the other lot gave me constipation, and the third lot gave me indigestion. In the end, I just thought to myself one day – fuck all of them! I'm over 80. I'm sick of people telling me what's good for me – I'll just take the ones I want, when I want. Since then I've never felt better…"

I wondered what all the *brainiac* neurologists, neuroscientists and pharmacologists would have made of this guy's *do-it-yourself* medication regime. I guessed that his neurologist didn't have the slightest idea of what was actually happening, and had presumed that the prescribed medication regime was an outstanding success. This was one of the ironies of the relationship that appeared to exist (or failed to exist) between some patients and their neurologists. There was often a big disconnect between what the neurologists thought was going on and what was actually going on. It led me to wonder whether this guy's neurologist regularly appeared at international conferences, heralding his particular cocktail of prescribed PD pharmaceuticals as a triumphant success, based upon case studies such as this octogenarian.

Interestingly, we had a couple of other people who were septuagenarians, and they too seemed to have a steely resolve that was completely unfazed by the PD that afflicted them. The interesting thing about these people was that they didn't have grandiose expectations from life – they didn't feel cheated by the disease and nor did they harbor any bitterness. These people had been through wars and other tragedies and, to them, having PD was just another item to add to the *life sucks – let's just get on with it* file. That is not to say that they didn't suffer from the disease –

they did. They just didn't seem (outwardly) to be fazed by it.

One couple who came in were a *Ma and Pa Kettle* duo from the country. Pa had to contend with PD, and he also had to contend with Ma telling him how to sit; how to walk and how good he was feeling. I asked Pa whether or not he had a deep-brain-stimulator device implanted. Out of earshot of Ma, he replied under his breath,

"Listen son, I get all the deep brain stimulation I can handle from listening to her nagging all day. The last thing I want is to have some doctor implant an FM radio in my brain to add to the fucking noise level. When you've had to listen to the same woman's nagging for 50 years, putting up with a bit of Parkinson's doesn't seem so bad by comparison…"

Ma either didn't hear Pa's uncharitable comments, or chose not to hear them, or had heard them so many times that she was immune. Either way, it was clear that Pa had an invaluable lifetime companion in Ma, who helped him get through his PD – or else applied her deep brain nagging therapy to comparatively lessen the effects of the conventional PD symptoms. Chalk up another medical miracle for The Lancet, or for Robert L. Ripley.

Another thing that impressed me about Ma and Pa Kettle was that Ma had been prepared to drive Pa in from the country, and subject him to an hour of in-car nagging in each direction, just to participate in our little research experiment. Ma looked like she had just finished milking a hundred cows by hand, and plowing a few hundred acres with an egg-beater, before making the journey, fully attired in her best floral dress. Even more extraordinary was the fact that, far from being put out, Ma and Pa thanked us for letting them participate in our research.

In my cynical engineering manner, whenever I spoke casually to the people who came in with PD, I always asked them why they had gone to all the trouble of helping out. As someone who refused to spend 30 seconds filling out a survey form, this willingness to contribute several hours of one's life to a research project intrigued me almost as much as the disease. Were these people coming in because they felt vulnerable? Or, perhaps, because they thought that we could help them? Were they expecting some sort of cure as a result of coming in? I always tried to be frank and told people at the outset that the most likely outcome from our research would be that we would just cross off another avenue of investigation and that would be it. The response I got from one of our septuagenarians, however, was quite moving, even to a cold-hearted, cynical, sarcastic engineer:

"No. No. I'm not expecting any sort of cure. It's too late for me to get any benefit out of all this stuff. I'm passed all of that. I've already had my life and I'm happy. But... you say to me that that the research you're doing is probably not that important. And then you asked me what it was like having Parkinson's. Well, let me tell you that it's a terrible, terrible thing. I've got family and friends to help look after me and I don't need to work. So I'm very lucky. But I wouldn't want this terrible thing that I've got to afflict another person if I thought that I could do anything in my power to stop it. And that's why I'm here today. Because I couldn't live with myself if I thought that I could have done something to stop this and I hadn't done it. That's why it's important for me to be here."

Some of the younger people with Parkinson's, whom we met, didn't have this same level of steely resolve. They felt very vulnerable, reticent, timid and, in some cases, just afraid of what the future held for them. It was also evident that many of them had not only been separated from their professional circles but also from their social circles – they were just plain isolated and presented with a degree of *aloneness* that one doesn't generally come across in day to day life.

The obvious question that had always been in the back of my mind, from the time we had commenced our research, was where were all these people with PD?

PD was such a commonly occurring disorder, and yet one hardly ever saw afflicted people in the street. In discussing this with others, I found that many people had an elderly relative, someplace, who had PD – but where were the rest? After all, one in five PD people were contracting the disease between the ages of 30 and 40. That meant at least one person in every thousand had young-onset PD – and where were they? The answer to this question, however, turned out to be somewhat disturbing.

Many of the more elderly sufferers of PD don't go out much and, while they have friends and family as carers, they at least have a reasonable quality of social life. As their disorder progresses, or as their carers get older and find it more difficult to care for them, many of the older sufferers go into nursing care facilities.

The ones that are most profoundly hit by PD, however, are the younger people, for whom visual appearance in the modern world is, sadly, an important (if not critical) aspect in terms of socializing. Young-onset sufferers are often self conscious about their flailing arm or about their tremor. The fact that it is difficult for some of them to even have normal facial expressions means that friends think that they are being cold, indifferent or aloof. People afflicted at an early age often find that they can no longer drive a car, so it is even harder for them to go out on their own and socialize. It is sometimes difficult for parents to play with their own children, and often they feel that their children will be embarrassed in front of school friends by the disconcerting movements of their PD.

Some sufferers find it difficult to do basic things like brushing their hair; tying up a necktie, or shaving. Frequently, carers, who are also partners, husbands or wives become exasperated because their spouse appears to become more and more untidy and they have to keep picking up after them.

Many younger people with PD find that their symptoms become so overwhelmingly disruptive that they can't maintain normal work after a few years, so they lose the social and professional networks that are an integral benefit of work. They also lose the sense of self-worth that comes from being a contributor. And, in the final analysis, they feel as though someone has pulled the rug out from under them and the plans that they have had for their lives.

Above all, from talking to our participants, it became clear that many people with PD had lost confidence in themselves and in going out at all, because of the idiosyncratic nature of both the disease and the medication. One of the more severely afflicted people that came to see us explained his problem as follows:

"When you see me now, I'm fully functional, and nobody would even think that that was anything wrong with me. I'm very high functioning when my medication is *on*. But, sometimes, I'm walking down the street and some of my fingers start twitching. I have to decide whether it's just stress or just a regular jitter or if it's the PD medication wearing off. My transitions can be very abrupt and very severe. If the medication goes *off*, I'm almost frozen and I can't do anything without help. People in the street look at you as if you're drunk or on drugs or something. It's hard to even get people to help you to take your medication. They don't understand. It makes it very frightening to go out on your own. It also means that you're constantly stressing out on whether or not to take medication at a particular time. People get annoyed with me because I'm so cranky. But I always feel stressed and on edge."

So, if nothing else came out of our research, at least we found out where many of the people with Parkinson's were. Many of them had lost the confidence to go out and socialize and, as their disorder progressed, even more had lost their independence. Isolation appeared to be a key issue, particularly with the younger sufferers. It seemed rather extraordinary that nearly one in every 200 people in some populations faced these sorts of problems and, yet, most of the others weren't even aware that a problem existed.

In many countries, regional support groups were often established by governments or as self-organized groupings, created by people who had PD themselves. The purpose of these groups was not only to provide support, advice and access to various resources, but also to endeavor to reduce the isolation that people with PD faced. The irony of all this, of course, was that the mainstream society from which many of these people were isolated, was not even aware of the support groups, much less the individuals who had the problems. When I asked one of our participants why she didn't become involved with one of her local support groups, it was made clear to me why even this was difficult:

"I don't want to mix with other people who have Parkinson's just because they have Parkinson's. It's my affliction, it's not my personal hobby or interest. Do you hang out with other people just because they're the same height or weight as you are? Or because they wear the same size shoes? Of course not. I feel isolated because I want to mix with my family – and with other people who share the same interests that I do – and all the people I've ever known don't have Parkinson's. That's why I feel like a bit of an outsider. People just don't seem to understand that – they want to lump us all together as though we're all the same because we have a particular disorder."

This comment did provide an interesting lesson in what should have been rather obvious. It also demonstrated why even well-meaning government based decisions sometimes had limited impact upon the lives of those whom they were intended to assist. It all seemed to be about the way we treated people with disorders. All the ones with Multiple Sclerosis can be put into one group and all the ones with Parkinson's into another; the ones with renal failure can go into yet another group – they'll all be happy together because they have one disease in common. They reality is that many of them have nothing whatsoever in common except for the fact that they have a particular disorder.

Of course, in practice, people with particular disorders generally have a specific range of needs in terms of professional advice and support. The mistake we make is to assume that the provision of these sorts of bureau services, important as they are, can extend to fixing the sorts of isolation problems that people with particular disorders face.

In the case of PD, even the basic supporting services in our state appeared to be poorly funded and, apparently, relative to other states, our state had done reasonably well. Nevertheless, in our state, people with PD only received a fraction of the funding that was made available to support other neurological disorders, such as Multiple Sclerosis, which was a significantly rarer affliction. As it turned out, while we were conducting our research, I had the opportunity to speak to one of our most senior state politicians about the level of funding made available to support people with PD, relative to other disorders. I was given an interesting *off-the-record* insight into the way funding operated at government level.

Essentially, I was told that governments didn't particularly care how much they spent each year in order to be seen to support a particular disorder, unless it became a visible election issue – generally these funding issues (as they pertained to a specific disorder) were so small as a fraction of a budget that they received little or no attention. The hard part was getting them into the budget in the first place. Beyond that, it appeared that once a disorder was funded, in terms of support, it was very unlikely that funding would ever be cut and highly likely, given sufficient lobbying, that regular increases to funding would occur. In our state, PD had received a small amount of funding but required a quantum leap in order to become of use to those who were afflicted by the disorder.

The argument that this particular politician made to me, in regard to PD funding, was that it never appeared on the radar. He too had an old aunt afflicted by PD but never thought about it beyond that. He wasn't even aware that it afflicted a large number of younger people. Ironically, in order to get PD onto the government radar, it was necessary to have a strong lobby group. In order to have a strong lobby group it was necessary to have a strong support group. In order to have a strong support group it was necessary to either already have government funding or else to have self-organized groups of volunteers. In the case of PD, the very nature of the disorder heightened isolation so, in effect, there was a *Catch-22* situation, and it was difficult to get a quantum leap in funding. This seemed to be a common problem all over the world.

In our state, a government/volunteer funded agency did its best to cope on funding that seemed remarkably meager relative to the scale of the problem that its clients faced. The newly-appointed director of our state-based organization turned out to be a pleasant fellow, who also, fortunately, had had extensive experience in the media in the United Kingdom. In forming a relationship with our state based agency, for our research program, it seemed to me that our university also had an obligation to do something in return for the support group.

It appeared to us that there was a case to be made for the university to form some sort of collaboration with the Parkinson's support group, and in having our university provide students in the areas of social and behavioral science to work with the group – for research projects; undergraduate work experience, and so on. This would provide a two-way benefit – with the students getting first-hand interaction with people at the coal face, and the support group potentially having access to a larger range of assistants. A formal relationship would also expose undergraduate students to the disorder and increase awareness overall.

In discussions with our local Parkinson's support group, we generally agreed that, given their current position, it would be unwise, in the short-term, to get involved in the bottomless money-pit of neuroscientific research. Rather, a focus instead upon the social requirements of the afflicted constituents would provide a far greater short-term impact, and create a sense of movement, involvement and inertia. It was much easier to communicate social outcomes and achievements to the media than it was to explain complex scientific ideas. Often, it was also the case that sufferers felt vulnerable and developed unrealistic expectations in terms of cures arising from neuroscientific research – and when the cures don't miraculously appear they become bitterly disappointed and annoyed that they have invested hope, time and money in them.

The director of the local PD support group appeared to agree with this hypothesis, and also restated the difficulty of getting complex research concepts into the media, whose primary interest was a 15-second snatch for the evening news. Social concepts were much easier to sell and would create a much greater level of leveraging for any monies that were expended.

As our relationship with the Parkinson's support group grew, and our understanding of its director's media prowess grew, I decided to invite him to present a keynote address at a conference I was organizing at the university. The topic of his address was on using the media to support not-for-profit organizations, in a world that was saturated with messages and requests for money. During his talk, he eloquently made the point that the *worthy cause* message simply didn't cut it with the public any more. There were thousands of genuinely *worthy causes* bombarding the media every second of every day, and people had just tuned out. In a world where everything is worthy, every minute of every day, then nothing appears worthy – it all becomes background noise. His contention was that, in order to get people's attention, a message had to be entertaining – importantly it had to be interesting or funny or both. People should want to listen and, if the message was to have any value, it had to be memorable enough for people to do something about it.

During our conference, the director of our state-based Parkinson's support group talked for almost an hour. He told jokes and amusing anecdotes and had the audience of over 130 people in fits of laughter. During the course of his talk, the subject of PD was only mentioned once, and for less than a minute – and yet, at the end of it all, no one left the session without a clear sense of the seriousness of the problem he was tackling.

Ironically, having seen the effectiveness of this approach, a few weeks later, I was talking to one of our Parkinson's participants, who brought up the subject of the new director of the support group. He was concerned that they should have appointed, in his words, *someone who would take the disease seriously.*

"What we needed was an eminent neurologist to run the group – not a comedian…"

I responded with,

"The last thing in the world that that a Parkinson's support group needs is an eminent neurologist to run it – unless the guy does stand-up comedy during his consultations. At the moment nobody is listening to you. *N o b o d y*. Not the public, not the politicians and not the media. You have a broken down building for a support headquarters and now they're planning to tear that down to put up a car park. I mean, Moses smell the roses, your message is just not getting out there. And the public is not going to listen to a neurologist – they just won't capture public attention. This guy has the potential to do something good and to get your message out there – he's funny; he's interesting, and he is a great communicator."

"I don't like the idea of someone making fun of a disease. It's not a laughing matter for me."

"I think you're missing the point. No one is making fun of a disease. This guy makes fun of himself. He's makes fun of life and he's getting a serious message out there in a way that makes people sit up and listen. When he presented at our conference, he was the fifth speaker on the day. Most of the people had difficulty staying awake for the first four. When he spoke, he had the audience mesmerized. If a neurologist had presented at that session, he would have ended up walking off the stage to the thunderous sound of his own footsteps. I think you're very lucky to have this guy, so give him a break – if it doesn't work out, then you can think about going back to a neurologist."

Over the coming weeks, coincidentally, the Parkinson's support group was also looking to hold their annual general meeting, and I graciously offered the conference facilities at our research institute, thinking that this was the least that we could do in recognition of their support. But, then, one day the phone rang and it was the Director of the Parkinson's support group:

"Hello…It's payback time."

"Payback time for what?" I asked.

"Payback time for you to make a presentation to our annual general meeting."

"Look," I said, with my mind still filled with thoughts of my great success at the young-onset PD group, "I'd really like to help you out but I really don't think that I'm qualified to discuss PD at your board meeting – in front of people who are world experts in the field yet."

"Look, you know as much about PD as I know about medical imaging and computer control of manufacturing systems – and you had me speak at those sorts of functions. All you have to be is funny and interesting."

"Alright, touché." What else could I possibly have said anyway? I owed this guy and he had me well and truly cornered. Little did this man know how unfunny and uninteresting we engineers could really be in mixed company. But, anyway, how much more of a fool could I possibly make of myself on this subject? Since starting this research, I'd humiliated myself in front of one my colleagues; I'd thoroughly embarrassed myself in front of the young-onset group, and looked like a complete pompous fool in front of the cosmetics assistant at the pharmacy. How much more risky could it be in giving a half hour lecture on a subject about which my knowledge was almost worthless – to a group of people, some of whom were leading neurologists in the field?

As the days ticked by, and we were less than a week out from the board meeting, I was still mulling over what I could possibly present to these people. The phone rang and it turned out to be the assistant from the PD support group:

"I'm just calling to finalize the arrangements for the board meeting next week. I'm sending out details of how the board members can get to the conference room in your building. I've got the room number and it looks like the room is on the second level – where is the elevator in your building?"

"Elevator? What elevator? It's a two storey building – we don't have an elevator."

"Well how are some of the members going to get up the stairs? Some of them are quite disabled as a result of their Parkinson's."

"Parkinson's? You didn't mention people on the board having Parkinson's. You told me it was a Parkinson's annual meeting."

"Well, what sort of people did you expect would be coming to a Parkinson's annual meeting?"

"To be honest, it never really crossed my mind. I guess I assumed that the board was made up of neurologists and government people, and so on."

"Well it is. But some of the people have PD. Anyway, they can't climb two flights of stairs. Do you have another room on the ground floor?"

"Other conference rooms? We don't have any other conference rooms in our building. The other conference rooms are in other parts of the university. They have their own cost centers. I would actually have to lease those from the university in order to book them."

"Well, we've already sent out notices telling people that the meeting will be at the university."

"Alright. Leave it with me and I'll see what I can find."

A few frantic phone calls later and I found another venue – a new lecture theatre – with an elevator. After significant groveling with the head of the department who managed the theatre, I convinced them that they should donate it to the PD cause for an afternoon, rather than charging their usual fee. I decided on telling them the truth about messing up the booking by forgetting to consider the elevator (or lack thereof) in our building. The honesty seemed to work, and the pack of lies that I had on hand to use if honesty had failed ultimately wasn't necessary. The lady in charge of the theatre even assured me that there was an elevator right outside the door.

A few days before the event, the lady from the PD support group called to thank me for reorganizing the venue.

"And this one has an elevator right in front of the door," I proudly proclaimed.

"That's excellent. Thank you for doing that for us. That's wonderful. And there are no steps inside the theatre to mess us up?"

"Steps? You didn't mention anything about steps inside the theatre before. It's a lecture theatre for Christ's sake. It's full of steps. It's like *Fiddler on the Roof.* It has one long staircase just going up, and one even longer coming down – and one going nowhere and just for show. It's a lecture theatre – it has to have steps."

"Well perhaps the people with Parkinson's who can't climb can just sit in the front row."

"Good idea. If you tell me how many people need front row seats, I'll see how many seats are there, and maybe we can get some more temporary ones in."

Now this already appeared to be an inauspicious beginning to making a presentation to the PD annual meeting, and there were still two full days to go, which left plenty of time for things to completely fall to pieces if necessary.

On the day of the meeting, I thought I had better call the lecture theatre booking officer just one more time to make sure that it was ok:

"Yes. I have it written down here. We have you fully booked in for this afternoon for the Parkinson's group. It'll be a very nice venue for them. They should be happy with it. Except for that darned elevator of course – hardly ever seems to be working these days."

"Is there another elevator in that building?"

"No. But people can always use the stairs if the elevator isn't walking – it's only four flights."

"Now listen to me," I said. "The whole reason for booking that lecture theatre was because I had a bunch of people who couldn't walk up two flights of stairs to our conference room, and now you're telling me that it's only four flights up to yours. And then, when they get there, they have even more stairs to go up in order to sit down."

"Well if you were concerned about it, you should have booked a room on the ground floor. That doesn't need an elevator and there are no stairs inside."

"You didn't tell me you had any rooms on the ground floor."

"That's because you didn't ask for venues on the ground floor. You asked for one with elevator access. That's the only large room we have with elevator access."

"Well didn't you realize that the reason I wanted it was because...Oh never mind. Do you have any rooms available on the ground floor for this afternoon?"

"Let me check...No. No. We don't. They were all booked out two weeks ago."

I couldn't quite understand how I had managed to survive for more than four decades without ever once paying the slightest bit of attention to the world's elevators and stairs and, now, they seemed to be haunting every part of every conversation for the past two weeks.

Miraculously, however, the elevator did happen to be working that day so that I could at least turn up for the event with head held high.

"Nice venue," someone commented as they greeted me when I walked in.

"Thank you. I chose it especially because of the elevator," I replied. "We always have to consider those people who can't climb stairs," I asserted proudly, as my nose doubled in length.

When I came to present at the session, I decided that it was pointless having the guileless leading the bewildered on the subject of PD. I thought that it would be better if the people who were there got a clear picture of what research went on in our university, in terms of the various sciences and technologies that pertained to PD. I also wanted to give them a hard-nosed view of what went on in research at an international level, and to remove all the smoke and mirrors and *goody-two-shoes* perceptions of the research and academic worlds. That is, to make sure that no one left the session with any delusions about the purpose of research or about prospects for impending miracle breakthroughs.

I presented the audience with a time-line containing just some of the various research paths that had been investigated from James Parkinson's original identification of the disorder (to the present day), and showed how, statistically, simply pumping money into research problems wouldn't necessarily make an enormous contribution to the time it took to solve them. I sensed that some of the audience didn't really like what they were hearing, and had been hoping for a more optimistic assessment. Needless to say, the obvious question presented itself:

"When do you think that they're going to cure this thing?"

I tried to be somewhat circumspect in my reply,

"It's not really my field, but from what I've read I don't personally believe that it is possible to even say at this point in time. And, it's probably even less appropriate for me to comment as an outsider to the field. What I can tell you, based upon my limited reading of what has been happening in the neurosciences, is that there appears to be no short-term prospect for a complete scientific solution because the current understanding of the brain is so limited. Scientists are still working with individual neurons and trying to extrapolate their behavior upwards to global brain function – that is not a trivial task – it may well be a bigger task than all the neuroscience that has gone on in the two centuries leading up to this. And, ironically, therefore, if a solution comes today, tomorrow or in a year, or ten years, it may well arrive fortuitously rather than scientifically – that is, by scientists stumbling across it well before they have a sufficient understanding of the brain to know why the solution works."

All of this seemed to evoke a stone-faced response, and I wasn't sure whether it was because I was perceived to be the cold, clinical engineer who thought diseases were no more serious an issue than a broken toaster or washing machine. I thought that I had better finish with something more positive:

"That having been said, scientists may alternatively find that incremental improvements in medication over the coming decade outstrip the urgency for an outright cure – because the medications may become so effective at treating the symptoms and because the side effects become so much less onerous. There is also a much greater business impetus for treating PD with life-long drugs than there is in curing it. To give you some insight, on their website, the Mayo Clinic in the US, for example, claims that the provision of PD drugs, in the US alone, costs six billion dollars a year – that probably equates to around 18 billion dollars a year worldwide. So you can imagine how much money pharmaceutical companies will be prepared to invest to come up with life-long medication solutions rather than outright cures. And, because of this investment, and because pharmaceutical companies are focused on continuous, small, short-term improvements, rather than revolutionary new treatment paradigms, they may well be like the tortoise and win out in the end."

I'm not sure that these sorts of comments were altogether welcomed, and I didn't have enough conviction to be burnt at the stake with them but, at least, they were my honest, ill-informed and uneducated opinions on the subject. They may have been naive (or even completely wrong, perish the thought) but they were my genuine thoughts – rather than the usual collection of spin-doctored research rhetoric used to attract research funding or media interest. I thought that these people had to put up with so much other shit in their lives that, at least, they deserved this much. After the session, one of the audience asked me the inevitable question that had clearly been inspired by media reporting of science:

"But what about stem-cells?"

Again, I found it difficult to come up with an answer that I thought would be palatable (or, for that matter, one which I even understood, given that I knew next to nothing about the field), so I decided to just tell them what I thought, with the same level of knowledge and passion that a taxi-driver uses to tell passengers how to solve world hunger, the Middle East peace crisis, and economic depression:

"As a complete outsider to the field, the science of stem-cells, appears to me, at least, to be the science of individual neurons. The brain is composed of billions of neurons, all with complex interconnections, most of which are not fully understood. To my way of thinking, a stem-cell is like a brick or a building block. So – ask yourself this – if you know how to make a brick, do you then automatically have the skills to build a cathedral? The skills required to understand how all the bricks fit together to form a cathedral are completely different. Now, add this complication to the whole stem-cell problem – specifically that we are expecting the stem-cells to build their own cathedral – and critically to know when to stop building – because if they don't know when to stop building then we are looking at the possibility of cells building tumors. All of this appears to me to be an enormous leap from making one stem-cell. And, from what I can see, the world of neuroscience doesn't appear to have those sorts of skills – yet. Now, they may be fortunate and discover that the stem-cells magically take care of the cathedral building for themselves, and they may magically know when to stop building – but, at this point, that seems to me to be a question of luck rather than science."

Another person with PD asked the logical follow up question:

"Well if it isn't simply about spending more money on research in the short term, then what can we do to accelerate research into a cure?"

Another annoyingly pertinent question to which I had no real answer. But then, I probably wasn't the only one and, if they were being truthful to themselves, even those who are genuinely committed within the field of research would struggle with a pathway forward. After all, the question was really about expediting serendipity. My off-the-cuff suggestion was as follows:

"Volunteer to participate in research. If you have the disease, then try and participate as much as you can in research. The greater the numbers of people that involve themselves in testing, and the greater the variety of people that are involved in testing, the more meaningful the results of any research investigation – and the more quickly that unproductive pathways can be eliminated. I think that, if you have PD, then there is probably nothing more productive or valuable that you could possibly do at this point in time."

8 ADDING UP THE SIGNIFICANCE

"...we may quote to one another with a chuckle the words of the Wise Statesman, lies, damned lies and statistics, still there are some easy figures which the simplest must understand but the astutest cannot wriggle out of ...These are the figures I have done my best to simplify and set intelligibly before you. I now leave the way clear for the wriggling."

J A Baines,

Parliamentary Representative in England

*Journal of the Royal Statistical Society **59** (1896), 38-118, pp87.*

A number of people have been credited with the famous statement about *lies, damned lies and statistics*. These include Leonard Henry Courtney (in 1895, in a speech on proportional representation in New York); J.A. Baines (quoting from Courtney in 1895); Benjamin Disraeli (who apparently never actually said it), and Mark Twain (who penned it in his autobiography in 1904, thinking he was quoting Disraeli, who apparently never actually said it). There is a supreme sense of irony in the fact that the statistics about the statement on *lies, damned lies and statistics* are themselves somewhat muddled within the statistics of history. There is also irony in the fact that many research outcomes are muddled within the very statistics that are used to scientifically substantiate those outcomes.

Whoever actually coined the phrase about *lies, damned lies and statistics,* inadvertently described, with remarkable accuracy, three basic tools that academics and researchers around the world sometimes employ to claw their way up the ladder of academic eminence. As a general principle of ethics, one hopes that scientific discoveries have been founded upon the third tool, although the first two are not altogether uncommon.

Before I tell you about the outcomes of our research program into Parkinson's Disease (PD), I need to fill you in on some of the harsher realities of what happens in the world of research. If you've read this far, you probably already have some insight into these, and you may have already worked out what a bitter, twisted person I am. Be that as it may, I need to again caution you that the land of research isn't the land of *sunshine and bananas* that outsiders believe it to be. The problem with research, as with everything else in life, is that it is based upon people – and people are people, whether they are undertaking research; running a large energy corporation or, for that matter, preaching an entire religion. So, the moral is that in order to interpret research outcomes, you also need to understand the realities of the research environment and the people within it.

I have already told you that it is very difficult, in the modern world, to assess the significance of any research outcomes, regardless of how eminent the originator and the research organization or university that generated them, and regardless of how eminent the publications in which they appear. No matter how many rules that bureaucrats apply in order to stamp out fraud, or to measure the significance of a piece of research, people being people, tend to find ways around them.

The most important lesson that we need to take from this is that the only real way that we have of assessing the impact of research is to wait, and wait, and wait. And, if after years and years, people are still talking and writing about a piece of research or, better still, if they are actually using it because it has been turned into a useful product (or a service or a treatment or a cure), then the work is deemed to have made an impact.

The problem with the *wait and wait and wait* approach is that it makes it very difficult for academic career climbers to plan their ascent, and to claw their way up, because it means that they may actually have to spend years, decades or even lifetimes without any recognition, reward or promotion. Those who wish to become eminent before their 40th birthday are then forced into either fortuitously making some earth-shattering scientific discovery, whilst in their 30s, or else in adopting the *lies, damned lies and statistics* approach to get a foothold on their upward climb. There is a strong case to be made that the research world has always been thus, and it is just that sophisticated search tools, such as the Internet, have just shone a light into this dark and mysterious realm – in so doing they have exposed its shortcomings and machinations, which are fundamentally born of human nature.

The purpose of the statement about the *lies, damned lies and statistics* was of course to highlight the fact that even the selective use of statistics, to justify an argument, is the same as using lies or damned lies. Nevertheless, correctly and ethically applied, statistics can provide some scientific measure of the value of research outcomes, particularly numerical ones. The problem is that even ethically presented research statistics need to be interpreted and debated by learned peers in order to avoid jumping to incorrect conclusions.

Unfortunately, universities and other research organizations around the world tend to get their core funding and competitive grants based upon previous research outcomes or, more accurately, on perceived previous outcomes. So, the more grandiose the claims, and the greater the overstatement, the greater the likelihood of getting core or competitive funding for further research.

One may well ask why all research claims aren't independently substantiated before anyone is permitted to derive benefit from them – however, in practice, such a process is both costly and complex, so many decisions are, by necessity, based upon a combination of perceived integrity, reputation and trust. In the majority of cases this is a well founded process. Unfortunately, this sometimes also means that decisions can be inadvertently based upon the careful marketing of scientific ideas.

Marketing is the art of using statistics in order to give people sufficient information to enable them to jump to the wrong conclusion. For example, we all know that, "*...contains 5% real fruit juice*" is the way that a marketing person would describe a product that contains *95% water*. For this reason, the marketing of research findings, and the statistics that are used to support the marketing, create serious problems for the researchers, the public, governments and funding bodies. Are the researchers telling us about the *5% real fruit juice* or about the *95% water*?

In universities and research institutions, there are two types of marketing that are employed. The first type is the one that the public sees, which is about selling simplistic *research breakthroughs* to the mass media. This is the one that helps to get the public on side – perhaps to have people donate money to a university or research institute, or to send their children to study there – or even to go as far as lobbying their politicians to increase the amount of funding allocated to such a *noble* cause. The second type of marketing is much more complicated and is the one that is used to sell the university to learnt peers by getting publications, citations and awards. This type of marketing helps the university to build up its core funding or to leverage its capacity to get competitive grants.

This brings us to the perceived need for research institutes and universities to make grandiose marketing claims about their *excellence* or *world leadership* in particular areas. Traditionally, universities and researchers didn't make such claims, and issues of excellence or leadership were left to the judgment of learnt and impartial outsiders. Unfortunately, these organizations discovered that the funding decisions, which supported research, weren't always made by learnt and impartial outsiders. Often, such decisions were made by politicians, bureaucrats and well-meaning benefactors, particularly when it came to large-scale funding. For these reasons, the smoke-and-mirrors marketing approach to research often worked far more effectively than the traditional approach – which was to actually be excellent and let other people work this out for themselves.

Research providers, in recent years, have also become smart enough to recognize that if they can get a research message out into the mass media, then the leveraging effect with government and other funding bodies is greatly enhanced. If researchers can get the message to the public that their organization is close to, say, a cure for a particular disease, then public pressure on government and other funding body representatives mounts to the extent where funding may be favorably skewed. This ties in with the more subtle form of marketing employed by research providers in order to leverage funding from government, industry and benefactorial bodies – that is, to politically position themselves or their staff in such a way that they directly influence the actual expenditure or grant allocation process.

As a general rule of thumb, the best way to determine how the research marketing game is played is to simply follow the money trail – that is, determine where all the research money comes from; find out who makes the decisions about where it is spent, and then find out where the money ultimately goes. If you take the trouble to do this, you might be mortified at what actually goes on in the world of research – and, then again, you might not – perhaps you would ascribe this to human nature.

Those that are involved in research at a senior level know all too well how the *game* is played. They either have to decide to check their morals in at the door when they come to work, and opt in to the *game*, or else work out a way to maintain their integrity and survive the *game*. Whichever way one looks at it, the *game* unfortunately hinges, to a large extent, upon the way in which research is marketed. I once heard an eminent researcher claim that he

"...never once came across a young medical researcher who entered the game without the intention and passion to do good for humanity..."

I could have added to this, that I have met very few senior researchers who got to where they were without by-passing the passion; the humanity and the intention of doing good – opting instead to just play the research game.

If you are outside the research community, then generally the only time you come across the marketing of research is in newspapers, the evening news or current affairs programs. And, what you tend to see is marketing spin – firstly, from the marketing departments in universities and research institutions and, secondly, from the media representatives. Institutional marketing experts convert raw research statistics into a form that is more *interesting* to media representatives – the media representatives subsequently turn the *interesting* information into a format which they believe to be *newsworthy* to their readers or viewers. Sometimes, what eventuates is a story that has no relationship whatsoever to the original research data. Often, the result is little more than a few seconds or minutes of noise in an evening news or current affairs program:

"University researchers have found a link between baldness in male rats and the consumption of peanuts..."

It is ironic that a news or current affairs program, whose lead-in story is about someone claiming to have been abducted by aliens, can be completely scorned at one level and yet, when the next story is one about a medical research breakthrough, the same program is treated as a reputable source of scientific information:

"It must be true because I saw a man in a white laboratory coat with a stethoscope - he had a test-tube in his hand and said that this was a scientific breakthrough…."

Sadly, not all of the media-reported research findings emanating from universities are seen as filler, and many vulnerable people take them very seriously – particularly in those instances where the research claims pertain to cures or treatments for serious diseases.

One of the advantages (or disadvantages) of being involved in engineering research is that the mass media never bothers to cover it. For one thing, the mass media doesn't understand engineering and has no capacity to turn it into filler material for news. For another, the journalists that I have spoken to tell me that engineering stories would be edited out even if the reporters could find a way to explain them in simple terms:

"…there's no human interest element – and human interest is what rates and sells newspapers…".

Being of no interest whatsoever to humans is an integral part of being an engineer, and it generally means that we don't have to concern ourselves with how engineering research outcomes are reported in the mass media – because they're not reported at all. In the case of our doctoral research program into PD, and its outcomes, a number of the people that we told about them surprisingly said, "that's very interesting…", which is something that we engineers seldom hear about anything that we do. So, I have decided to tell you about our outcomes and what we decided to do with them in the hope that you might also say "that's very interesting…"

Of course, after all that I've just told you, you should now be wearing a cynical expression on your face and treat what follows with skepticism. The point in telling you about our research outcomes is so that you can see what sort of things can come out of research and so that perhaps you may also say,

"Gee, I don't know why everyone says that engineers are so boring…"

Ultimately, any significance (if there is any significance) that can be ascribed to our findings can only materialize after others have independently reproduced the work or have done something worthwhile with it. And, that may be days, months or years from now – or possibly never. So, with your most cynical expression now installed on your face, let's begin.

First of all, I have already told you (and told you …and told you – because repetition is good) that our objective was to study the auditory brainstem responses (ABRs) of a group of people with PD and to compare these against those derived from people with no history of neurological disorders. I have reproduced the typical diagram of an ABR (presented earlier) which is a modified version of one prepared by the American Speech and Hearing Association (ASHA). This is shown as Figure 8.1.

The squiggly waveform depicts voltage as a function of time, as measured from a couple of electrodes placed behind each ear. The waveform shows the brain's electrical response to sound and is actually the average (ensemble) of the brain's response to hundreds of short auditory stimuli (clicks). Just to recap – the peaks on the squiggly waveform are called waves. The timing of the waves are referred to as latencies.

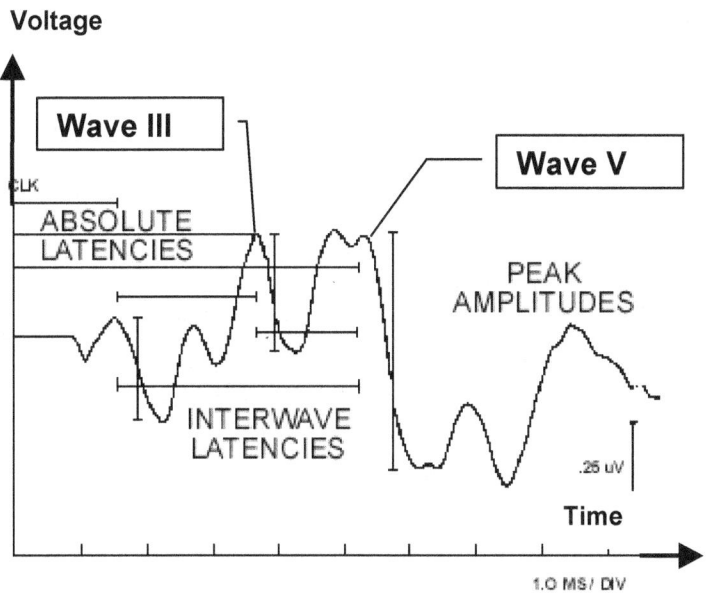

Figure 8.1 – Typical ABR (Modified from the American Speech and Hearing Association)

In our research, we were particularly interested in the amplitudes of the peaks, particularly of Waves III and V. We were also interested in the latencies of Waves III and V. We wanted to determine whether any of these factors varied with the presence of PD and, for that matter, whether the ABRs varied with Parkinson's medication. A change in either the wave amplitudes or peaks (or both) would also result in a change in ABR waveform morphology (i.e., waveform shape). So, in simple terms, we wanted to know if the ABR waveform shape was affected by PD or the associated medication levels.

From the results of our experiments with a control group, and a group of people with PD, we effectively wanted to create a table of results, as shown in Table 8.1.

Experiment	ABR Wave III Amplitude	ABR Wave V Amplitude	ABR Wave III Latency	ABR Wave V Latency	Webster's Mobility	Core Body Temp.
PD Patients Morning "On"						
PD Patients Afternoon "Off"						
PD Patients Afternoon "On"						
Control Group						

Table 8.1 – Results Matrix

A simple table, such as this, would enable us to answer five basic questions in regard to the participating groups, and in regard to PD:

Question 1:

Was the ABR of an unmedicated Parkinson's participant fundamentally different to that of an unmedicated control group member?

Question 2:

Did the ABR of a Parkinson's participant change with medication level?

Question 3:

Was the ABR of a medicated Parkinson's participant fundamentally different to that of an unmedicated control group member?

Question 4:

Was there a relationship between various ABR parameters and participant mobility?

Question5:

Did the ABR of a Parkinson's participant vary with time of day (i.e., diurnal factors)?

Given the difficulty in recruiting participants, and because of the time involved in organizing and conducting the tests, we ultimately had 15 control group participants and 15 participants with PD.

Of the 15 participants with PD, one was determined to have a severe manifestation of the disorder and was excluded from subsequent testing – primarily because we were concerned with having a severely afflicted person present in their medication *off* state without appropriate support staff. A second participant with PD had been implanted with a *Deep Brain Stimulator* (DBS) device and, because it was difficult to obtain noise-free measurements, was also excluded. This left a total of 13 participants, mildly afflicted with PD, who went through the entire test regime.

Table 8.1 looks relatively straightforward but one needs to remember that, for each participant, and for each test, two sets of ABRs had to be recorded for each ear. For each Parkinson's participant, a mobility test had to be undertaken to determine their mobility at the time of the ABR test. So, for each participant, the process took a considerable amount of time for each session. And, with travel time to and from the institute, each Parkinson's participant gave up more than half a day to contribute to each session.

The results that arose from the experiments proved to be extremely interesting. In answer to Question 1 (above), in all 13 cases, the morphology (shape) of the ABR waveform of an unmedicated Parkinson's participant was markedly different to the morphology of the ABR waveform of a control group participant. Not only that, but the amplitudes of Waves III and V were markedly lower for unmedicated Parkinson's people than they were for the control group. In other words, in comparing a mildly-afflicted person with PD to one with no history of neurological disorders, we found a significant difference between ABR shapes and amplitudes. Also interesting was the fact that there was no significant difference in the latencies.

The answer to the second question also proved to be profound. We discovered that when patients took their Parkinson's medication (and the participants we tested used a variety of different medications, primarily Levodopa), their ABR waveforms went back to *normal* (so to speak) as soon as they were fully *on*. So, in answer to the third question, our experiments indicated that a person with PD, who was fully medicated and highly functional (in terms of their measured mobility), had a similar ABR to a person with no history of neurological disorders.

This led us to an answer to the fourth question. Our results indicated that there appeared to be a correlation between participant mobility and the amplitude of Waves III and V in their ABR response. The poorer the mobility, the lower the amplitudes of Waves III and V.

In regard to the fifth question, and the impact of diurnal factors on ABR, we found no evidence of any correlation.

In summary, the *good* news (from a research perspective, not from an afflicted person's perspective) was that there appeared to be a strong correlation between some of the auditory brainstem response (ABR) parameters (particularly amplitude) and the level of impairment associated with PD. Moreover, our results tended to show the variation of the ABR with medication levels.

So, what could we conclude from this? Firstly, it appeared from our experimental data that there was a research case to be made for further exploring the ABR as a potential diagnostic tool for PD. There was also a case to be made for pursuing the ABR as a potential means of measuring medication effectiveness. Notwithstanding this, we had to recognize that even though the raw data appeared to be compelling, we had only used small sample group. Statistically, one would say that the likelihood of the results being a *freak* occurrence would be small but one would nevertheless need to have the experiments independently assessed elsewhere to be sure that what we discovered was a valid trend.

In terms of statistics, the problem with small sample sizes is that when one averages numbers, the average of a small sample may not reflect the average of the entire population. For example, if one measured the height of a random sample of ten people, this might give a figure of 1.7 meters. If one averaged the height of a random sample of 1000 people, then the average might be 1.73 meters. A random sample of 100,000 people might provide an average height of 1.74 meters, and so on.

There are both traditional and modern mathematical/statistical techniques that can be employed to assess the likelihood of numbers, derived from a small sample, being an accurate reflection of the total population. In our research, we subjected the results to several different statistical tests – the first was an analysis of variance (ANOVA); the second was known as *Student's t-test* (a traditional statistical test, which has some limitations), and the third was referred to as a *permutation analysis* (the modern day, computer-based technique that provides a more comprehensive analysis of the data).

Our analysis showed that, in a statistical sense, the likelihood of us being correct in saying that ABR amplitudes were affected by PD and Parkinson's medication was better than 99.95%. In statistical terms, this is referred to as a significant result. Taking a more mature research outlook, one would ideally like the whole process to be repeated with a different control group and different Parkinson's group in order to be fully comfortable.

What our results didn't show, and what we didn't test for, was whether the ABRs of people with PD were different to the ABRs of people who had similar disorders, such as Multiple System Atrophy (MSA). In our case, for a number of reasons, not the least of which was the difficulty of recruiting people with MSA for experiments, and managing them in a non medical research institute, it was decided not to do this as part of the doctoral research. However, this would have been the logical follow-on step in an ongoing research process.

The other thing that we didn't do was to measure the ABRs of severely afflicted Parkinson's patients to see if they were even further removed from the control group than the mildly afflicted ones we tested. As I have already mentioned, we didn't do this because we didn't have the facilities or staff to handle people severely afflicted with PD while they were in the medication *off* state.

So, in summary, we got a great deal of research satisfaction out of a set of results that looked promising and experimentally supported an idea that seemed altogether sensible from an engineering perspective if not a medical one. But, the next question was, where to from here? Our major priority was in ensuring that our doctoral candidate completed his PhD dissertation and had it internationally examined, so that he we could get some form of independent assessment of the work, and so that he could move forward with his life and career.

The bigger issue for the rest of us was what to do with the outcomes and whether it was worth us pursuing the project any further, particularly given that, as an engineering-based research institute, we didn't really even have a mandate to be involved in this sort of work in the first place.

There were really only a few options open to us. The first was to seek additional research funding to undertake a much more comprehensive clinical testing study, which would include a larger numbers of participants; people with MSA, and people severely afflicted with PD. The second option was to seek a commercial route, on the assumption that a practical, low-cost testing device could ultimately be manufactured based upon the outcomes of our research – this would have required us to establish a relationship with an entrepreneur who could provide seed funding for development and more clinical studies, and who could access venture capital for product development and commercialization.

At this point you need to understand that if we wanted to just pursue the research further, then the potential pathways forward were limited. Firstly, our own institute or university could have agreed to provide internal funds to pursue the work. This is not a common practice in universities and research institutes because the general system is one which encourages researchers to pursue competitive grants for research. A competitive grant is a sum of money, derived from government, industry or benefactorial organizations, which is used to set up a project – for example, to hire a postdoctoral researcher; pay postgraduate research scholarships; fund equipment, and so on.

The concept of a competitive grant is an attractive one, particularly if one feels that one is actually competitive. In our case, we didn't feel that we could put forward a competitive case for competitive funding in a field in which we didn't have a research and publications track record. In engineering, one way or another I'd always managed to fall into grant monies (competitive and otherwise) because, after a while, the process is fairly routine and funding isn't such a big issue. In this case, it was all about starting over with no background; no track record, and no imprimatur of a relevant research institute to bolster an application. Nevertheless, as the principal research supervisor for the project, it was incumbent upon me to go through all the various mechanisms and cross them off the list before finally calling it a day.

In going through the various options, it became clear that in order to pursue funding, we would be competing against grant applications from (what were perceived to be) the world's most prestigious neuroscientific/medical research organizations.

Years ago, in my naïve, innocent youth, I would have been in awe of such organizations because I would have assumed that, by reputation alone, they were doing extraordinary research. However, in my dotage, I had at least come to the realization that there were no such things as prestigious institutions – after all, an institution is just a collection of individuals working on their research projects. And, regardless of the institution, some of the individuals can be brilliant; some can be good; some can be ok, some can be mediocre and some just plain bad. Nevertheless, the ratios of brilliant to good to ok to mediocre to bad are obviously much higher in places that have genuinely earned their prestige. And then of course for the leaders there are the essential resources for moving forward in non-theoretical fields – internal research funding; critical research mass/expertise; research infrastructure; technical support; global research connections; ability to attract the smartest students from around the world, and so on.

In scouring the Internet, I did discover that one thing that large *prestige* research organizations seemed to have in common was an uncanny ability to get their senior staff onto scientific advisory committees, sitting in judgment on competitive grant applications and funding policies. And, even more uncanny was the fact that, when I searched the Internet to follow the money trail, I discovered that many of their home institutions had also been remarkably successful in getting *competitive* grants from the same bodies. A remarkable coincidence to be sure. Not a conflict of interest by any means – rather, an expedient convergence of interests.

In choosing to follow the research money trail for any given field, therefore, one quickly learns why research tends to trundle along in one direction for decades or even centuries, even when that direction is not particularly fruitful. The inertia is enormous. Universities and research institutes have many millions of dollars tied up in infrastructure and staffing that is geared towards a particular path of research investigation. The last thing that the head of a research organization wants to hear is that another path of investigation is proving to be more fruitful, and that they don't have the capacity to get onto it. The harsh reality is that although researchers present themselves to the public as selfless humanitarians, behind the scenes, research is big business – not necessarily a profit-making business, but a big business all the same.

At a global level, in a particular field of endeavor, there may be hundreds of millions of dollars and thousands of staff and research students committed to a particular path of investigation. It simply isn't practical to slam on the brakes on one path and move to another path overnight.

As a result of the enormous inertia in the research system, mechanisms are either consciously or subconsciously put in place to preserve the status quo, and therefore change tends to be very slow. It is a very naïve young researcher that believes that the research system welcomes radical ideas that challenge existing paradigms – despite the fact that the image of radical change is what is generally presented to the public through the media.

With this as background, you may get some insight into why there would have been little benefit in us pursuing ongoing funding for our project through conventional competitive grant routes. Fundamentally, it was a case of us opening up an alternative research path and then presenting this to research heavyweights who were already busy fighting to fund their own research paths. That is not to imply in any way that our research path would have been any better or any more fruitful than what was already in place – it just would have been different – and that is a very difficult (if not impossible) proposition to sell in the business of research when one is an outsider to a particular field.

In terms of the business of business, in order to move our project forward we would have had to find an entrepreneur who was willing to provide seed funding and develop a business case that could be put to a venture capitalist. The problem with this was that it would be difficult to protect the intellectual property emanating from our research, as it currently stood. On the other hand, if we had actually been able to use the findings to produce a novel *wearable* device that people with Parkinson's could use over the course of a day (to evaluate the performance of their medication), then that could potentially have been protected. However, this would require further investment and clinical trials which would, in turn, need to be funded by someone. And, venture capitalists generally don't fund things where there is no core intellectual property that has been protected. So, you can see where this is headed – it is a *Catch 22* scenario – no intellectual property, no venture capital – no venture capital no intellectual property.

As if by divine intervention from one of those far away cows, just as I was busily crossing off the possible routes for extending our research project, an email came to me through the university system. The email said that the university was negotiating benefactorial funding to pursue research into PD – and that they wanted to find out what researchers were currently doing in the area, and what sorts of projects should be funded. I was somewhat surprised by the timing of this announcement and even more surprised that the university had managed to track down a benefactorial body to fund research in the field. We had already gone through both the national and international list of potential funding bodies and had crossed them all off the list – in most cases we decided that we would be uncompetitive and, in the remaining cases, we determined that the bodies simply didn't have enough resources to provide any significant funds. So, who was putting up the money to fund this research?

It turned out that after my presentation to the annual meeting of our state-based PD support organization, they had considered the possibility of funding research programs, and had been in touch with our university to see if they could form an alliance. As the PD organization was small, and our university was relatively small, there appeared to be a good fit. And, if the university was prepared to play ball and show some commitment, the PD organization indicated that they would fund one or two postgraduate research scholarships to get things going.

It did cross my mind to question whether the Parkinson's organization had decided to form an alliance with our university because of my involvement in our research program or despite my involvement in it. From an egotistical perspective, I chose to believe the former rather than the latter, and decided not to question the good fortune, lest I find out the true reason.

Within a few weeks, the university had collected a summary of the various research projects that were under way and a list of potential projects for support, including ours. One day the phone rang and it was the director of the PD organization. He told me that there was to be a meeting between himself; a member of the University Council, and the head of the university's alumni and development department to discuss what to pursue in terms of research. Would I be interested in coming along to put in my two cents worth? This was intended to be a very simple question but it had significant implications for us. In agreeing to attend such a meeting, and in providing an opinion, I would have no choice but to withdraw our project from the potential list of ones to be funded. It would have been, in my view, completely unethical to have expressed an opinion on directions while having an active grant application.

In the high stakes world of the *research game*, when big research players are involved in grant committees, such a direct conflict of interest would normally be resolved by the rather bizarre practice of the affected party *leaving the room* while his or her grant application was discussed – as if that would make the slightest bit of difference to the bias that was intrinsically present in the committee. However, I wasn't in the *high stakes research game* and had little interest in joining it.

The decision I had to make was, in my view, a very simple one. Research grants come and go but people rarely get the opportunity to contribute to shaping processes that can develop a higher sense of purpose. This appeared to be one such process that, if properly managed, could provide a worthwhile outcome for people who had PD, rather than just for the research grant recipients. I agreed to participate in the meeting and, in so doing, effectively killed off the last available funding option for extending our own research project. In the final analysis, it seemed to me that if something was going to happen with the outcomes of our project, then it was going to happen anyway. As none of the logical follow up paths appeared very logical from our perspective, the best approach seemed to be to let the future of our project take care of itself and to concern ourselves with getting the best outcome for the people who needed it more than we did.

In attending the meeting, I again strongly put forward my argument that there was little benefit in a small charitable organization getting involved in the funding of neuroscientific research in the field of PD. A couple of research scholarships, one way or another, were not likely to make the difference between finding the cure for PD and not finding it. It appeared to me to be a case of *a mere drop in the ocean*, particularly when many of the organizations already involved in neuroscientific research were enormously wealthy North American research institutes, whose individual turnover was hundreds of times the size of our local PD support organization.

My argument was that we should be looking to find research projects that were of direct social benefit to the Parkinson's community in the short-term. This would enable people to more actively participate in the research process and to see tangible outcomes. If people could see tangible benefits in the short-term projects, then they were more likely to develop the trust necessary to pursue longer-term objectives. With scientific research, on the other hand, its very nature tends to exclude the community that contributes to that research through participation – it is very difficult to report back intermediate research findings and, often, it is difficult to convincingly explain their significance.

The meeting went on for a couple of hours and, once again, either because of my arguments or despite them, it was agreed that the first two projects pursued would be in the areas of social and behavioral science. The research would look towards improving the lot of those who already had the disease and all the social problems that it created. It was also agreed that, as part of the alliance, the university would engage in joint fundraising activities with the PD organization, with the objective of funding further collaborative research on an ongoing basis.

When I left the meeting, it occurred to me that the outcomes of this meeting appeared to be far better for the local PD community than anything I would have envisaged only days earlier. The PD support group would fund research that would directly impact upon its constituents, and the university would also throw some weight behind the cause. It appeared to me to be the best leveraging that the Parkinson's community would get for its contribution to the alliance.

So, you see, ultimately, life and research are all about those far away cows, and about making the best of shorter-term decisions – and about letting the longer-term ones take care of themselves. Some people view research in terms of getting a nice neat set of experimental statistics that they can claim will revolutionize the world. In our case, our research outcome appeared to be that, by stumbling our way through one research program, a series of coincidental events would lead to an outcome that was probably better, for the people who mattered the most in this process, than what we might have achieved with our own research or with other research grants. And, only time would tell what would actually happen with the statistics of our research.

9 A FORK IN THE ROAD

If you have managed to read this far, you are probably beginning to wonder when you are going to get to the part of the book with all the melodrama, tension and angst. If you have fanned through the book, you've probably also started to think to yourself that there don't appear to be enough pages left for any of these things to build up to a dramatic crescendo. If you think this way, then you're probably one of many people who have had their life's expectations of the professional world completely warped by fictional novels, movie and television melodrama. If you have read this far, you will also have worked out that, as far as engineers are concerned, the only times we use words such as *melodrama*, *tension* and *angst* are in completing crossword puzzles.

However, before you begin to yearn for the melodramatic in your life, and in your reading, perhaps you need to consider the consequences of having the sorts of zealots, who are portrayed as *passionate* professionals in books, movies and television shows, working for you in real life. Consider going into a real hospital emergency room, only to find all the medicos thumping their fists in rage and yelling:

"Get me those goddamn test results - stat!"

Would you seriously want someone like that making decisions about a life-threatening condition, or about some toxic medication that he was about to inject into you? Or, what would you think about being in an aircraft that was making a rapid descent, only to hear the sound of an angry co-pilot's voice emerging from the cockpit:

"Damn you all to hell! You're not fit to be flying this aircraft. I'm taking command!"

The reason that you don't often hear these things in real life is because real professionals generally don't behave in the sort of hyped-up, melodramatic manner in which artists portray them in books, movies and television shows. In over two decades as a professional engineer, I can honestly say that the only time I've ever heard a professional engineer thump their fist and ask for anything *stat* was when ordering a glass of beer at a bar. And, if I ever have the misfortune of going into a hospital emergency room, I'd kind of hope that the medical people in there remained calm, quiet and disconnected, and saved their fist-thumping zeal for their golf games.

An important part of being a professional is in understanding that work is work and life is life, and the two don't necessarily have a lot in common. To this end, I can say that, without exception, all the most intelligent, professional and productive people that I have ever encountered have always been the ones who have been able to disconnect themselves, their personal biases and their careers, from their decision making. And, yes, it is still possible for professional people to be very passionate about something and to remain impartial and detached. In other words, it is possible to be passionate without being a zealot. So, for those who have to go into real hospital emergency rooms, or to fly on real aircraft, it is comforting to know that professional decisions are generally based on calm and impartial assessments of facts, rather than melodrama.

As far as research is concerned, a good rule of thumb is to always put one's faith in the cynics and never the zealots. Good research is only partly about trying to move things forward – it is equally about trying to understand the truth – sometimes, the truth is hidden and even experimental results don't show it in its entirety. Often this means that researchers need to disprove things, or to try to find out why good experimental results may have some fundamental flaws in them. The good researchers are cynical and reserved about their research outcomes, and always ask *"why is it so?"*. The zealots welcome, without question, experimental results that substantiate their theories, and so they have an innate capacity to provide an animated *yippee* or *eureka* that makes for good storytelling.

For those who choose to write books, or make movies or television shows about professionals, zealots with *yippee* or *eureka* discoveries are naturally always far more interesting and persuasive than detached cynics. Let's face it – nobody wins a Pulitzer prize for writing a story about a mousy accountant who just does his job for forty years, and nobody wins an Academy Award for accurately portraying a physicist who just sits in an office for decades, quietly doing his calculations and getting nowhere. A lack of melodrama tends to diminish the weight of a message in the mind of a reader or viewer, and so artistic license often has to be employed. Artists, being emotional people (relative to we engineers), tend to think that scientific people are the same as they are – and so that is the way they interpret them in art. In bringing out the *real professional*, artists generally create a cartoon character that one rarely encounters in real life.

In order to satisfy those of you who have an artistic bent, or would have preferred something more melodramatic, I would have dearly loved for you to have gotten up to this chapter, and for me to have exclaimed:

"Goddamn it! It was the "banana and bag of peanuts" all along. We've found the cure! It's been staring us in the face all along! How could we be so blind? Why didn't we just see it earlier? My God! Let's get this thing out there and start curing people – stat!"

Unfortunately, such a convenient and well-packaged ending simply wasn't possible with our research project, and therefore you are not going to get one of those conventionally happy endings to finish this particular story – just a whole bunch of things to go away and think about for yourselves about Parkinson's Disease (PD). And you should think about these things seriously because one in every two hundred of you that read this book either already have, or will contract, PD at some stage in your lives. If you think that this makes the disease just an outside chance, then consider whether or not you would invest a dollar on a lottery ticket at the same odds.

There is something even more disturbing to think about in terms of the statistics as they pertain to PD – some of you reading this now will be thinking *"thank God I don't have to worry about it…"* and, yet, unbeknown to you and your doctor, may already be lurking the disease – unnoticeable and undiagnosable – perhaps for another several years. As I have already told you, PD is a very slowly progressive disorder that doesn't appear to play favorites.

As a hypochondriac, in order to allay my own fears, I reviewed the scientific literature to find out whether any other neurotic, 40-something engineers, who wash and wax their cars twice a week, have ever contracted PD – so far none have turned up, and I have to take solace in that. The rest of you can make up your own meaningless rules for why you won't be one of the people who get it.

Having provided you with these warnings about both the disease and the anticlimactic ending to this story, we can now move on with the conclusion.

In terms of our research project, I would like to have told you that its outcome had set the neuroscientific research world on fire – but, it didn't. I would like to have told you that what we did was going to have an enormous impact on the lives of people with PD – but, it probably won't – at least, not directly. I would like to have told you, in the spirit of Horace Mann's 1859 statement,

"Be ashamed to die until you have won some victory for humanity…"

that our research had won some victory for humanity – but, it hasn't yet. The end result is that you will have to satisfy yourselves with some contrived and Pyrrhic victories that I have created to assuage my own ego, and to bring to some finality my excursion upon the hackneyed and clichéd *road less travelled*.

To begin with, you need to understand what happens with research findings after a project has been completed. This, and where elephants go to die, are two of the great mysteries of the universe. We do know, however, where research projects begin their *afterlife*. First of all, research findings can be published in research theses, or in the innumerable scientific journals, for other people to read and use. Sometimes, other scientists read them, use them and create other findings which are also published and used. So, the original author can get some satisfaction from knowing that his or her findings have been formally cited and used by peers – hopefully for some ultimately valuable end purpose.

Each research paper or thesis effectively documents one possible link in a chain between the discovery of a problem and the discovery of its solution. Only a few, amongst an entire myriad of links, are critical ones, and all the others are there because they are an integral part of the process of elimination that leads to the critical ones. For this reason, when many research findings are published, they live out their retirement years on dusty library shelves or in the bowels of cyberspace, for months, years, or even forever, without being used by anyone.

As I am writing this, it is premature, in a research sense, to tell you what value our research would ultimately have or, indeed, if it would ever have any value at all, other than contributing to the process of elimination. I can tell you, on a more positive note, that our university did end up forming an alliance with the local Parkinson's support group, and that they did commence a process of collaborative research – specifically, in looking at a range of serious social issues that confront people who have PD. The outcomes of these will hopefully have some far more direct, shorter-term benefits for the people who have to endure the disorder. So, that was one collateral outcome of our research.

Our university and our local Parkinson's support group also got together in terms of fundraising, and in terms of locally raising the profile of the disorder. This too was a small victory for those who have the disease in our state. I only discovered that the formal alliance had occurred when I received an invitation to attend a combined university / PD fundraising art exhibition – or, as we engineers prefer to call such an event, a *framed wallpaper* exhibition. We engineers generally don't get invited to many things (certainly not for a second occasion, at any rate), so it seemed to be a good idea to accept.

Prior to receiving my invitation to the *framed wallpaper* exhibit, my last memorable visit to an art gallery had been almost two decades earlier, when I had visited the Guggenheim Museum, and wherein I had managed to set a record in viewing the entire gallery in under 15 minutes. A great achievement in the annals of engineering if not art.

"How did you find the Guggenheim?" people would ask.

"Walked up Fifth Avenue and there it was," I would reply.

"No, I meant weren't you impressed with the scope of the artwork?"

"All I can say is that it's a pity that they had to subsidize the entry fee with all those Campbell's Soup commercials over the walls."

"Those aren't commercials, they're art," people would tell me, while rolling their eyes in disbelief.

"And the difference between those and a Campbell's Soup billboard on a freeway would be what?" I would rhetorically enquire.

Usually, this comment would attract one of those condescending *engineering barbarians* looks that people with an interest in *framed wallpaper* give to us engineers. It would also terminate any further discussion on the fine arts. But, baiting artistic types with poisonous barbs is one of the few joys that we engineers derive from life (apart from baiting medicos), so please do not deny us such small pleasures. As far as this upcoming exhibition was concerned, however, I had decided to be on my best engineering behavior, given that it was for a good cause. I therefore cautioned myself to count to ten before issuing any poisonous engineering barbs at this affair.

When I arrived at the art gallery, I discovered that it was already cram packed with hundreds of people.

"This is your program for the exhibition," said someone near the entrance, as she handed me a few sheets of paper. "All the artists are listed here."

"*One-two-three-four-five-six-seven-eight-nine-ten*," I counted to myself before responding. "Oh, how nice. I see you've also included a phone number for each artist so that we can call them at any time," I remarked with the engineering sarcasm machinery on full.

"No. Those aren't phone numbers – those are the prices," remarked the lady with an incredulous and confused look on her face. "Would you like a drink?"

"Are the drinks on the same price scales as the art works?"

"No. The drinks are free."

"Good. Then I'll take two."

As I was directed to the front of the crowded gallery, I went past one of the artists next to her exhibit.

"Is there anything I can help you with in regard to my work?" She asked.

"*One-two-three-four-five-six-seven-eight-nine-ten*," I counted. Yes. Yes there is. What sort of art would you recommend to blend in with pale olive colored walls?"

Again, I received one of those confused and incredulous looks that artistic types give to us engineers. I decided that I ought to break the ice on this conversation, as it clearly wasn't going at all well:

"While you're thinking of an answer to that question, I might just go and help myself to some drinks."

As I got to the drinks area, I fortunately bumped into a fellow engineer.

"And are you an art aficionado?" I enquired.

"Yes. As a matter of fact, I am," he replied.

"So, how do you tell what is good art and what isn't?"

"It's fairly elementary if you're as cultured and refined as I am. You simply take the price tag for a painting, and then you divide the price by the surface area of the painting and the number of colors in it. For example, this painting costs $25,000 and has a surface area of two square meters. It also has about 20 colors in it. That gives me a result of 625. This other painting costs $21,000, has a surface area of one square meter, and has 12 colors in it. That gives me a result of 1750," he said, looking at his calculator.

"So, the $21,000 painting is almost three times better art than the $25,000 painting," he concluded.

"That's fantastic," I said. "So that's all there is to being artistically sensitive, cultured and refined?"

"That's all there is to it. Anyone can do it, even an engineer. All you need is a work of art, a price tag and a pocket calculator," he replied.

This was another victory that I had derived from taking *the road less travelled* – acquiring a detailed appreciation of fine art. From now on, whenever anyone asked me what I thought of a piece of art, I would ask them how much they paid for it and divide that by the area and the number of colors. This business of refined cultural awareness was a lot easier than I had ever imagined. And, with this newfound engineering approach to art appreciation, I didn't even have to be distracted by the aesthetics of a painting – I could just perform a cold, clinical engineering calculation in order to truly appreciate what the artist had in mind.

The other thing that I learnt from being at the art exhibition was that people found the fact that I was involved in PD to be interesting. This was quite unusual for an engineer.

"And what do you do for work?" Asked one lady.

"Actually, I'm an engi… – actually, I have been undertaking important research into Parkinson's Disease," I replied.

"Oh, that must be so interesting," she remarked.

"Yes. Yes it is. Particularly, the engineering aspects of it that we were looking …."

"Excuse me, sorry to interrupt you there, but I think I just saw someone that I know. I'll be right back a little later after I talk to them."

"*One-two-three-four-five-six-seven-eight-nine-ten* – take your time…I've got all night," I said outside of her hearing range, as she sped off.

So, another important lesson was derived from my foray into the world of Parkinson's research. No matter how you introduce anything relating to the word *engineer* or *engineering*, the *Easter Island Syndrome* response will always be precisely the same.

Shortly after this demoralizing encounter and lesson, a blonde lady came up to me to congratulate me for organizing the event. As it turned out, I had met this lady several times before at various other functions, and she was a well known target of many jokes in the circles in which she operated. She did mean well, however, and had somehow convinced herself that I was the instigator of the charity event. It appeared that the more I tried to explain to her that I had nothing whatsoever to do with the event or the fundraising, the more she was convinced that I had:

"Oh you're just being modest," she said. "I'm sure this whole thing has got your name all over it. I think it's wonderful that you're involved in Parkinson's research. Actually, my boyfriend is over there. He's in a very similar area of research."

"And what area is that?" I asked.

"Liver cancer. Is that similar to Parkinson's Disease?" she enquired.

Unfortunately, a couple of milliseconds before she had come up with this priceless response, I had just taken a mouthful of champagne which began spraying out through my nostrils and bubbling its way up through my ears. There was no time to count up to ten this time. Somehow, while trying to stop the explosion of laughter that was building up inside, I managed to cough out,

"Almost identical. Liver. Brain. I'm sure they're all connected. There's just so much we don't know isn't there?"

"Mmm. That's right. Mmm. It's so important to have the research isn't it?" she replied authoritatively.

"That was just a rhetorical question. You don't actually need to answer it right now. Excuse me, but I think I just saw someone that I know over there. They probably need my advice on assessing an art work – we engineers are very good at that sort of thing. We live for our art. I'll be right back a little later."

I hope that you recognize this incident as another important milestone outcome along *the road less travelled*. Quite possibly the first time in history that an engineer has been able to apply the *"...I think I just saw someone that I know over there – I'll be right back a little later"* line.

As I was about to leave the event, having acquired all the artistic appreciation that I could endure for one evening, another lady came up to me and asked,

"Do you remember me?"

I responded with, "No. Should I?"

"I was there when you presented at the young Parkinson's group a few months ago."

"Oh, sorry – I didn't recognize you. Do you have Parkinson's Disease?" I asked, still trying to work out who she was.

"No. But you sure looked like you had it when they finished with you," she responded with a smirk. "The boys gave you a harder time than you expected, did they?"

"Not really," I lied. "Just another average day in the world of research. No more or less humiliating – ...well, maybe a teensy bit more humiliating."

"Hope that it all worked out for you in the end."

"It did, thank you," I replied as I left. And, as far as the research was concerned, it had.

As I left the art exhibition that evening, at the back of my mind, I could see the *on-ramp* leading back to the *engineering freeway*, and further away from the *road less travelled.* The art exhibition appeared to be the end of the excursion.

A few days later, however, the telephone rang and the caller turned out to be one of our Parkinson's research participants.

"I just wanted to call you to thank you and your research student for the kind way in which you treated my wife and I whenever we came in. I'm actually in the process of writing you a letter to thank your research student formally."

"That's very nice of you, but there's really no need for you to do that. You've already done an enormous amount for us just by participating in our research. Anyway, I get paid for what I do, and if you say anything nice about our research student in writing, he'll only get a big head."

"No, I wanted to thank you properly. And, in the letter, I'm also including details about how I first noticed that I had the disease; and how it affects me – and how I explained what was happening to me – to my family. It might be important for you to understand that."

Despite my assurance that it wasn't necessary to send a formal thank you, sure enough, a few days later, the letter arrived and, in part, read as follows:

"…Enclosed is a note that I sent to my family and friends in the hope that they will continue to be understanding and not to worry about me so much. My carer is my wife of 51 years and she is wonderful.

I would say that my experience of Parkinson's has been better than other sufferers that I have met or spoken to. I have occasional spells of depression and anxiety but overall am managing reasonably well.

…The work you are doing is very important to us. Please thank your research student for being so pleasant and helpful to my wife and I.

…My main concern is the constant awareness that I am not able to make commitments or communicate properly while on the tightrope of medication. Parkinson pain is not severe but the discomfort is distracting. The digestive process…this is probably the most dangerous problem – I have difficulty swallowing – very untidy whilst eating. The real situation is that the whole muscular system is not working and coordination is very poor. …I have a magnificent John Cleese walk, which I try to limit to my wife's enjoyment. I also have quite a lot of involuntary movements which are exciting and unpredictable.

…I am very lucky to have a disease which can be treated by the drug Levodopa, with the help of many other ancillary drugs.

…There is no cure for Parkinson's, but many people have lived with it for 25 years or more. This will mean that I can get old and grumpy.

I am lucky – I am happy with my life and intend to continue to be a bloody nuisance…."

The letter, though perhaps unintentionally so, was both powerful and moving. It is a rare thing in life for even rich and healthy people to formally acknowledge that they are either happy or lucky. And, yet, here was this man who was, seemingly, neither rich nor healthy proclaiming himself to be both happy and lucky. His letter gave me pause to think back to old Sister Kevin, and her far away cows with the long horns.

That *far away cows have long horns* was really just an old Irish nun's Gaelic way of saying that the grass is always greener on the other side of the fence. And, more importantly, to not go looking for those far away things at the expense of happiness and living, because those far away things sometimes appear better than they really are.

The letter also led me to recall a conversation I had had some months earlier with one of the young-onset Parkinson's research participants, while we were waiting to set up for one of our tests.

"Do you think they're ever going to cure this thing? Do you think I'll ever be able to *get my life back*?" He asked.

"It's not my area of specialization and I'd just be speculating. You'd really need to ask a neuroscientist that question. What I can tell you with absolute certainty is that nobody is doing research into the area of *getting your life back* – they're just doing research into removing the symptoms of a disease – and that is not the same thing and you need to understand that. As far as getting rid of the symptoms is concerned, I'm guessing, because I don't really know, that the pharmaceuticals will end up giving you a significant improvement in your life long before you see a cure, just because of the amount of money involved in the development and commercialization of a cure. And, can I now also ask you a hypothetical question, instead?"

"Sure."

"Supposing, hypothetically, that rather than being an engineer, I was the world's greatest neuroscientist, and that I had read every piece of research on the subject of Parkinson's Disease. Supposing, then, I told you today that we were never, ever, ever going to find a cure for Parkinson's Disease. And that you believed my prognosis. What would you do today?"

After a pause, he replied, "I'm not really sure. I suppose I would have to sit down and think about it. I would have to work out how I could be making the most of every single day in my life, given where I was physically, and how I could enjoy every day to the best of my ability – knowing that things were never going to be better than they are today."

"That's a very interesting answer you've given, isn't it? Do you see the supreme irony in what you are saying and doing?" I queried.

"No, I'm not with you," he replied.

"Well, if I follow your reasoning through to its logical conclusion, I see it this way. Currently you have Parkinson's Disease and you're not as happy as you think you might otherwise be – because every day the disease seems to have taken something more away from you. However, somewhere, in the back of your mind, you're harboring a hope that one day there'll be a cure, and then all those things that have been taken will be returned to you – and you'll be happier because you'll *get your life back*. But, if today, I were to tell you that there was no hope of ever being cured, and that none of those things that have been taken will ever be returned, then you tell me that you would take stock of your life, and do something to make yourself happier than you are now. In other words, that you would actually be happier today if I gave you no hope than if I gave you some hope."

Just as I had finished saying this, I realized that I had really overstepped my mark with this whole conversation, and that I should have kept my mouth shut. It wasn't for me to go and make such a comment, and it had nothing to do with our research. I was also sure that I had made the guy angry and was about to be yelled at and told that I didn't understand his problem at all. Surprisingly, however, after a pause, the response I got was one of agreement:

"I think that's probably right. That is a very good point – and that makes me very nervous. Nobody's ever put it in those terms before. I've never really thought about it that way. That is a very disturbing thing you've given me to think about. And, I guess it's not something I ever really wanted to think about."

And, in truth, at the same moment that he made his realization, I also realized that this was indeed a very disturbing thing about research, life and diseases. Research has an intrinsic ability to improve the quality of our lives, but it also creates the illusion of those far away cows, that sometimes prevents us from making the best of what we currently have – because there is always the mirage of something intangibly better in the distance.

It would have been very easy then for us to have just dismissed the more mature sufferers that we met with PD as having a basis for greater contentment than the young-onset sufferers. Granted, the mature ones didn't have to work or pay mortgages, or to raise children. Some of the symptoms of PD also coincided with the symptoms of age, so they were not as pronounced in more elderly sufferers. Given this, the young-onset sufferers genuinely had been dealt a bad hand because far more had been taken away from them. But this line of reasoning would also have served a great injustice to some of the older PD sufferers. Their quiet acceptance of the problem and their understanding that science probably wouldn't be able to provide a rescue (for them) within their lifetimes had instilled them with a greater sense of purpose, and with a wisdom about how to handle PD, and the rest of their lives.

Notwithstanding this, having seen what PD could do, and to such large numbers of people, led me to hope that one day soon someone would find a better remedy than the treatments that currently exist. Perhaps a herbalist with a *banana and bag of peanuts* cure; or a pharmaceutical company with a lifelong pill that will make them even more billions of dollars; or a neuroscientist with a stem-cell – or perhaps even a naturopath, slapping a couple of dead fish over the tops of people's heads. But, on those occasions when I thought about the people who already had PD, I also realized that for many of them, a cure would be a far away cow. At best it would remove the symptoms but it would never reverse the hands of time and turn them back into the people that they were before they contracted the disease. And, if the truth be told, reversing the hands of time was one of the far away cows that many of them were in search of.

And that was probably the most significant thing that I learnt from our research.

In deference to old Sister Kevin (wherever she may now be), and her wisdom and philosophy on far away cows, and in deference to those who have PD, it would be unwise of me to conclude without quoting from something apropos. So, I have extracted part of a letter from Paul to the Corinthians, which I believe is as relevant to Sister Kevin and her far away cows as it is to this discussion, and as it was two thousand years ago:

> *In all things we suffer tribulation – but we be not anguished, or distressed;*
>
> *We be made poor – but we lack nothing;*
>
> *We suffer persecution – but we be not forsaken;*
>
> *We be made low – but we be not confounded;*
>
> *We be cast down, but we perish not.*

Anyway, you've probably heard enough from me on all this moist-eyed-bumpkin stuff. As an extremely busy engineer, I had to take the on-ramp from the *road less travelled*, back on to the *engineering freeway* and back to the important issues in life. I consulted my diary to see what critical engineering issues had been neglected during my foray onto that *road less travelled*. What vital diary entries needed my professional engineering attention? And there it was:

"Change cat's flea collar."

Yes. It was going to be another very busy and fulfilling week in the world of engineering.

ABOUT THE AUTHOR

Dario Toncich was born in Melbourne Australia in 1960 and graduated, with honors in Electrical Engineering, from the University of Melbourne in 1983. His industry based research led to a Master of Engineering (by Research) from SIT and a PhD from SUT. Since that time, he has held industrial, academic and research leadership positions, and has been involved in numerous research and development programs. In 1988, Dr. Toncich was appointed as the foundation research manager for the (then) recently established Key Centre for Computer Integrated Manufacture (CIM). In 1996, when the Centre was expanded into an industrial research institute (IRIS), he went on to become the research leader in automation and control; subsequently headed the Institute's postgraduate research and coursework programs, and contributed towards its strategic planning activities. In 2006, IRIS became one of Australia's longest established industry-oriented research and development centers, having celebrated its 21st anniversary.

Dr. Toncich has authored and coauthored a number of research papers in his field. He has also contributed towards several federal reviews of national research policy and expenditure. His views on industry research and development have been cited in government reviews and editorialized in Business Review Weekly. Dr. Toncich has supervised 22 Doctoral and Master's (by research) candidates to successful completion, and has authored five text books, including one on postgraduate research, which has been adopted by numerous universities and research institutes as their training text for research students. His field of research and Doctoral supervision has been in the areas of automation and control, with emphasis on feedback signals and signature analysis for both industrial and biomedical devices. Dr. Toncich's views and papers on higher education and research practice have been cited by governments and universities and appeared regularly in Campus Review. In 2007 he was appointed as the Project Manager for the University-wide research degrees admissions project at Monash University and in 2010 he worked as the Research Performance Analyst for the Office of the Senior Deputy Vice Chancellor and Deputy Vice Chancellor Research at Monash University, in the Research Strategy Unit. Dario Toncich also acts as an advisor on university research performance assessment and benchmarking with consulting firms.